Original French edition: "ECOUTE TON CORPS - ton plus grand
ami sur la Terre" first printing: 1987.
CAN ISBN 978-2-920932-00-5

Copyright © 1989 by Lise Bourbeau
Third edition/ Second Printing
National library of Canada
Bibliothèque et Archives nationales du Québec
ISBN 978-2-920932-02-9

Distributor
Lotus Brands Inc.
P.O. Box 325
Twin Lakes, WI
53181 USA
Tel: 414-889-8501; Fax: 414-889-8591

Publisher
Les Editions E.T.C. Inc.
1102 Boul. La Salette
Saint-Jerome (Quebec)
J5L 2J7   Canada
Tel: 450-431-5336; Fax: 450-431-0991
Email: info@leseditionsetc.com
www.leseditionsetc.com

Printed in Canada

LISE BOURBEAU

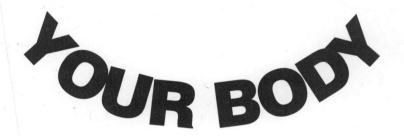

LISTEN TO
your best friend on Earth
YOUR BODY

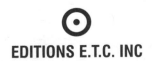

EDITIONS E.T.C. INC

ACKNOWLEDGMENTS

From the bottom of my heart, I gratefully acknowledge all those who trusted me enough to encourage me in writing this book. My deepest thanks go to the following people for the expertise and efficiency each has contributed toward the realization of this book: Odette Pelletier, Sylvie Besnard, Gail Masters, Bette Davies and Norma Connolly.

My most sincere thanks to you, dear reader, for acknowledging this book and sharing the information and philosophies you will now encounter between its covers. Thank you for your help in spreading a message of love everywhere on earth.

I dedicate this book particularly to my parents, brothers and sisters who, above all else, taught me how to love unconditionally by always accepting me as I am.

With Love,

Lise Bourbeau

LISE BOURBEAU

CONTENTS

FOREWORD

This book has been written especially for you. By venturing into its pages, you have consciously made a decision to improve the quality of your life.

For whatever reason you opened this book, be assured that throughout its pages you and I will become friends on your journey of transformation. As a friend, I will do everything I can to guide you and to help you discover your boundless inner blessings.

Hopefully, you have chosen to read this book because you've made the valuable decision to finally become the master of your life. In order to empower yourself to do so, we must work together. I will provide the methodology and simple guidelines; you will enter the process with a pure heart, an open mind and your full attention. Only you can apply these principles in your life. By following the steps as they are presented to you and by doing the exercises at the end of each chapter, you will greatly increase the odds of reaping the rewards of happiness and success beyond anything you've ever imagined, in every area of your life.

The contents of this book are the result of over 25 years of extensive research, study and personal observation. Having put these methods into practice in my own life, I have enjoyed tremendous happiness and personal fulfillment. Through my work, I have been able to help thousands of individuals transform their lives. Now I want to share my ideas with you. Together we will explore the Great Universal Laws of Life and enjoy the dynamic results that are only found on the path of personal discovery.

Take my hand and embark on the journey of your life - literally! May it be an amazing and enlightening one!

PART ONE:

THE GREAT UNIVERSAL LAWS OF LIFE

CHAPTER 1

A COMMON PURPOSE

Have you ever stopped to ask yourself what you are doing on this planet? Why are you here? What is your purpose? The answer is simply... TO EVOLVE, TO GROW. We are here to grow as individuals and grow collectively.

As manifestations of Universal Energy, as living things, once we stop growing, we die. Look around you - flowers and trees, birds and insects, plants and animals of every kind are growing and expressing themselves as living things. Once they stop, they die. As human beings, full expression of our growth happens on a soul level. The seed of the Divine Life Force is planted in the soul of every human being, thus, our sole purpose is our "soul purpose"!

In every religion, the fundamental truths are LOVE and FAITH. Being human, we become entangled in our problems, complicating our lives, throwing ourselves off the path and losing touch with these two simple truths. Jesus taught us that unconditional love for ourselves and for each other is the light that will keep our vision clear, allowing us to clearly see our path in life.

Once a human being has learned to love himself and others unconditionally, he will have mastered the material world and found inner peace and true fulfillment. We are all manifestations of God's pure love and energy.

Remember that the earth itself is a living entity. In Quantum Theory, we are tied to the earth and to each other on a cellular level. Physicists have known for many years that energy is indestructible and boundless. Our individual energy field, or life force, is interchangeable with everything and everyone around us, just as other fields interact with ours. In taking personal responsibility for our spiritual growth, we contribute to the growth of others and to the growth and harmony of our own planet. Each of us must take responsibility for purifying himself on every level - physically, emotionally, mentally and spiritually. Only in this way are we able to contribute to the harmony that is a critical element in our individual and collective prosperity.

Throughout this book, you will be given tools that will help you become MASTER OF YOUR LIFE. As you develop faith and love of yourself, you will radiate a powerful, positive energy that will transform everyone and everything around you. The chain of humanity is only as strong as its weakest link - do your part to give it strength.

As I am sure you are well aware, our world is in chaos. The pharmaceutical companies are thriving, hospitals, prisons and mental hospitals are overcrowded, crime and human atrocities are at an all-time high. There is an angst that permeates the planet. It is being absorbed by each of us and it affects each of us on a cellular level. We feel overpowered, saturated with negativity and utterly helpless to do anything about our own state of affairs, let alone the state of the world. You must take your eyes off what is happening outside of you and take a moment to look inward.

I know you are telling yourself "It sounds so easy, but I find it very difficult to look inside myself. I am afraid of what I might find." This fear has been programmed in your subconscious mind from past experiences on the material level, from your parents and from society in general. The point is, it has been programmed and has undermined the state of bliss that we are born into naturally - the supreme happiness that is our birthright. The universe creates us in happiness and love. If we have lost that state for whatever reason, we can find it again. IT IS OUR NATURAL STATE TO BE HAPPY AND TO GROW BY VIRTUE OF BEING ALIVE.

Do not be afraid to look inside yourself - you will find your inner power (which we will refer as your inner God from now on). Only by finding Him and befriending Him will you have all the strength you will need to accomplish what it is you desire, become master of your own life.

NOW you are living the most precious moment of all and the future depends on what you think or do NOW. Whatever happened in the past to cause you to feel unhappy and unfulfilled now, leave it in the past but learn from it. Then is then and now is <u>now</u>.

Within each of us is the seed of the Divine, of God's love and perfection. It need only be acknowledged, nurtured and allowed to grow until its beauty radiates and touches everything and everyone around you. You have a direct line to all that is good and pure - an umbilical cord to the Universal Source. By the time you reach the end of this book, you will become comfortable and familiar with your inner God, your source.

If you are a beginner on the path to personal growth, you may experience some distress and some discomfort on the physical and emotional levels. You might have the impression that your very foundation is crumbling as you let go of your old programming. It is only an illusion. You are ridding yourself of the shackles of the past - letting go of emotional baggage and preconceived ideas. YOU ARE BECOMING FREE! Once you learn to trust, to have faith in the process, you will let go of the fear and learn to love.

Regardless of the number of seminars you attend, self-help books you read, courses you take or the amount of time you spend thinking about the personal development process, YOU MUST ACT! Only through conscious action and repetition will you achieve your goals, intensifying your purification and growth. Remember, you are REPROGRAMMING your subconscious mind. The subconscious mind only understands ACTION!

For example, a glass of dirty water to which clean water is continually added, will eventually become a glass of clean water. The dirty water is displaced by the clean water. By reading about pouring clean water into the glass or by merely thinking about it, you will not have clean water. You will continue to have dirty water. ONLY BY DOING WILL YOU GET RESULTS! As you pour the clean water in, you will slowly but surely see results. Persist and it will pay off! You will get the results you are looking for if you remind yourself constantly that you are making progress.

Once you have made the decision to nurture your own seed, your essence, and take action, you will be amazed how quickly it will grow toward the light and the freedom that exists beyond the darkness of the soil in which it has been planted. Any pain experienced as you struggle through the soil will be temporary. If the pain becomes intense, it means you are resisting and refusing to "let go" or abandon old programming. You have everything to gain and nothing to lose. The more you resist, the more the pain will persist. You will soon feel the warmth of your love and the brightness of your inner light. LET GO AND LET GROW!

As an example of what can happen in everyday life, perhaps you have developed a sore on your body. In applying peroxide or some other ointment, you know that there will be temporary pain which indicates the healing is taking place. The same applies to your inner healing.

Remember that nothing can exist without having been imagined, dreamed or thought of. Creativity is the human being's greatest power. We are the only species, animal, vegetable or mineral, that can consciously create our own reality. As you enter into and persevere throughout the growth process, remain MINDFUL and understand that the only reality there is, exists in the inner realm. All else is illusion. Before becoming visible, everything is created in the invisible. Stay conscious of this truth at all times and you will become master of your own destiny.

Taking responsibility for your own growth will put you in direct alignment with The Divine Law and accelerate the process. The only reason you have not accomplished what you have wanted to in your life thus far is because you did not BELIEVE it was possible.

You did not have FAITH. One of the greatest mistakes we make as human beings is failing to accept this power. REMEMBER, thoughts are energy! Once your thoughts are clear, you will be able to manifest, to create whatever you want. This is a fundamental law of physics. The energy created by clear thought becomes actual, physical energy, to be molded into RESULTS.

Of primary importance is the realization that the subconscious reacts to ALL of your thoughts, therefore, if your mental processes are muddled and confused, the subconscious will also be confused and unable to manifest your desires.

CLEARLY define and visualize your desires, nurture them and make them grow strong! How discouraging to think that everything that happens to you is caused by outside influence. Imagine! If you feel others are responsible for your unhappiness, you will have to wait until they do something about it in order for you to be happy! If you are sick and blame someone or something outside yourself (whether you are blaming heredity or the weather, or whatever) you will have to be patient and wait until these outside influences change before you can be healthy! Are you ready and willing to wait this long? Do you like feeling powerless? Doesn't it make more sense to create your own health and your own life?

Take responsibility for your life NOW - know that THIS IN-STANT YOU CAN CHANGE YOUR LIFE...YOURSELF! You CAN learn to see the cup as half full rather than half empty! Once you learn to live from your heart instead of from your head, you will see through the eyes of love - you will see beauty and goodness all around you. Can you imagine feeling "in love with life" at all times?

Reality is what you perceive it to be - what you perceive as the truth will become your truth. Be selective with what you feed your mind. Take a minute to visualize yourself in a joyful scene and your body will feel happiness. Now see yourself as being lonely, your body will feel sadness. In an instant you changed your life. Train yourself to see beauty beyond ugliness, love beyond criticism. Being spiritual is to see love (GOD) and beauty everywhere, in everything and everyone..

By becoming reacquainted with your true self, the shell of your personality (or ego) will fall away and you will no longer need to define yourself by what others have perceived you to be. In more familiar terms, you will have "found yourself"...your true self. The facade that was once your ego will be changed. It will no longer be an obstacle in your life and YOU WILL BE FREE TO BE YOU!

CHAPTER 1 EXERCISES

I strongly recommend that you pay close attention to the exercises at the end of each chapter. Proceed with sincerity and positive anticipation and you will be rewarded with rapid results!

Take a sheet of paper and write down everything you can remember doing IN THE PAST WEEK in the following categories:

» What have you done just for yourself that made you feel good or brought you happiness?

» What did you do for others? What motivated you in each instance?

» List everyone who said or did something that made you feel criticized or judged. Then make a list of the situations in which you found yourself criticizing or judging others. How did you feel? Do you see the relationship between the two?

» Repeat the following affirmation whenever you are alone with your thoughts until you feel you have accepted and let go of the above situations. Then go on to Chapter 2.

I AM A MANIFESTATION OF THE DIVINE, I AM GOD AND I CREATE WHATEVER I DESIRE. KNOWING THIS, I FEEL A GREAT INNER STRENGTH AND A PROFOUND INNER PEACE.

CHAPTER 2

WHOLE MIND INTEGRATION

Having completed the exercises at the end of Chapter One, I'm sure you realized how often you are doing things unconsciously in your everyday life. You probably also realized that you could not remember the majority of your words and actions. How many times during the exercises did you find you had done things for others that you really didn't want to do? If you're like most people, you are living unconsciously. Don't worry about it.

Studies indicate that the average human being is 90% unconscious (only 10% conscious) of what they do, say, think and feel. Surprising, isn't it? Which means that you use 90% of your time per day acting, talking and thinking unconsciously. We will try together to modify your state of unconsciousness because becoming aware of what we feel, think, say or do is instrumental in getting what we want out of life.

The SUBCONSCIOUS MIND is situated in the solar plexus region, between your heart and your navel. It is directly in tune with your emotional body. I'm sure you are familiar with the phrases "gut reaction" and "gut instinct". The solar plexus is instantly reactive in any given situation - it is aligned with the subconscious mind and will react before your conscious mind has time to think.

Interestingly enough, the subconscious mind is like a computer. It can register up to 10,000 messages a day. Because it takes in data verbatim, it does not differentiate between correct and incorrect information - everything is undisputed fact. From the time of your conception and throughout your life, everything that is said, seen, heard and perceived by your senses has been registered.

Here is an example of the capabilities of the subconscious mind: As you travel to work, it absorbs every billboard, every passerby, even the names of every street you pass. Every sound, sight and smell is dutifully recorded. It is the duty of your subconscious mind to act as a buffer for the conscious mind. For the conscious mind to absorb and register all of this information would be overwhelming. It would be impossible to try and assimilate even a fraction of it.

The subconscious mind understands only the images that are reflected in your mind. That's why, when someone says "I don't want to have cancer", a picture is formed in the subconscious mind of someone who is dying of cancer. This person is unconsciously creating a cancer. Instead, she should visualize what she wants by saying "I want to be healthy". The subconscious mind will then relate to an image of a healthy body. REMEMBER: The subconscious mind does not understand positive or negative WORDS, only the IMAGES. When you imagine what you don't want, the image in your mind is of exactly that but without the "don't".

The subconscious mind does not reason: it accepts everything in the same way a computer accepts data. You can only retrieve what has been inputted. If you were to ask a computer the solution to three times four (3x4) when your intention was to find the solution to four times four (4x4), it will inevitably answer twelve (12) because it cannot guess that you made a mistake. It accepts orders as they are given. Likewise your subconscious mind registers every bit of information that has been inputted - and you function accordingly. You are constantly being fed information that may or may not be useful to you. How many times have you read an advertisement for a product, glanced at a billboard or watched a television commercial without being aware of consciously doing so? This information was being absorbed by your subconscious mind -the same process used in HYPNOSIS! Suddenly you find yourself in a supermarket with a strong desire to purchase that product, not realizing that you have been kind of hypnotized into it!

Most of us have no idea what vast quantities of information we register and to what degree we respond to this information. It is very important for you to be more conscious of what you allow into your subconscious mind. The subconscious can only help you to manifest what it has been fed. If you do not take some control of that information, what will be manifested will be chaos.

Continuously entertaining fears or surrounding yourself with negative people and situations will cause your subconscious mind to know only negativity - and that's what will continue to manifest in your life. An act as seemingly innocent as leaving your radio on while you are driving fills your subconscious with bad news and you become worried and fearful without understanding why!

Your subconscious mind reacts to the most recent information it receives on a given subject. For example: imagine your subconscious mind is a taxi driver and your thought is the passenger. It asks the driver to go to 123 First Street. He heads in that direction according to the information given him. Minutes later you decide you are in error and need to get to 456 Tenth Street instead. The driver will have to change direction. Like the taxi driver, your subconscious mind reacts to the most recent information. You must understand that your subconscious mind must be given clear directions in order for you to get where you want to go. Like the taxi driver, the subconscious mind, having been given a number of different instructions, will become impatient and demand "Make up your mind!" ONCE YOUR SUBCONSCIOUS MIND SEES THAT YOUR DIRECTION IS CLEAR, YOU WILL GET TO YOUR DESTINATION MUCH FASTER.

Here is another example: You have decided to move next year to a beautiful house by the water. You think a lot about that house - you imagine every detail, you visualize it. It is important to know that your subconscious mind understands only the pictures that go with the words you use. Visualize it clearly and consistently so that it becomes so real in your mind that you could almost move into the visualization. It is almost assured that within the year, you will have that house. How? With what money? Do not focus on the obstacles - focus on the goal and act in that direction - you will reap in proportion to what you sow. Give your subconscious mind the order and let it guide you. You will get there the same way you do when you tell your taxi driver where you want to go. There is no need to tell him how to get there, he knows the best way.

Do not let the opinions of others influence you. It is best not to reveal your intentions to others, as it triggers reactions in them based on their own obstacles. These obstacles, as others will express them to you, will be heard by your subconscious mind and will become obstacles to you on your own path. You will begin to doubt your dreams. "Maybe I'm moving too fast" or "I will never have enough money to do this" or "I don't really deserve this" (for whatever reason - I'm sure you can come up with many). As you let these doubts seep into your subconscious mind, you will interrupt the momentum. As you create obstacles, your subconscious mind interprets as follows: "We will not have this result". Having lost momentum, it is possible to gain it back, just by reprogramming the subconscious with positive and motivating thoughts consistently. THE SUBCONSCIOUS MIND REACTS ONLY TO ITS MOST RECENT INFORMATION.

Human beings are continuously inconsistent in their thinking. We must learn to increase our capacity for concentration - to focus - in order to get where we are going.

START NOW! Visualize your ideal life. Would you like to be surrounded by love? ...to have better relationships with your family? ...to have a job that you find fulfilling? Your subconscious mind will help you achieve anything you desire. It is up to you to learn to work with it and to learn to harness the power that it has. TAKE ACTION! If you are unhappy with your job, take the time to visualize yourself finding the perfect job for you - get excited about it and feel it as if it were real. Put your subconscious to work on manifesting your perfect job by understanding what that job "feels like". If you become too analytical about what you require of your perfect job (i.e.: a certain type of boss, a specific location, etc.), you will minimize your chances of finding it. It will minimize your options by giving your subconscious mind fewer places to look. It would be like telling your taxi driver which streets to take to get you to your destination... it could take much longer and cost you more. Trust that he will use his knowledge and expertise to get you there in the most expedient manner.

Your subconscious mind is connected directly to your superconscious mind, which has an overview of all the options available to you and the quickest route to them. Give your subconscious mind a picture of the finished product and place no emphasis on "how to get there". It will know the way.

Do you desire a mate? Visualize yourself with someone who makes you happy - someone who is "just the right fit". Again, if you limit your thinking to "this eye color, that height, no snoring, no dentures, etc.", you will limit your chances of finding someone who is a fantastic match for you -someone who brings out the best in you. That person is the finished product! Statistically, in an average-sized North American city, there are at least 10,000 people of the opposite sex who are compatible with you.

The SUPERCONSCIOUS MIND is also known as your "Divine Self", or your "GOD SELF". It has a handle on the big picture - your past and future lives, your life plan and which road you need to follow in order to achieve divine perfection. So, when you ask, desire or think you have a real need, make your request to your subconscious mind, but be sure to ask your superconscious mind to let you know if what you want is really beneficial to you. If it is not, you will receive a signal to let go - it will also lead you to a more desirable outcome.

Perhaps the house near the water is not of greatest benefit to you -there may be something that will serve your needs and desires much better. Usually, within a month of your making the request to your superconscious mind, you will experience something radical that will give you a very clear indication as to whether or not your desire was appropriately beneficial - and an alternate will present itself to you.

How reassuring to know that this power is within you and that it is directly connected to the great Universal Power, to the entire cosmos and to the superconscious mind of every human being! Everything is connected - all energy is one!

YOUR SUPERCONSCIOUS MIND IS YOUR BEST FRIEND! It is always there to guide and support you, every hour, every minute of your life. Learn to communicate with it, build a relationship with it, and it will never let you down. It may be a good idea to give it a name - something that will not remind you of anything or anyone else or that will not conjure up memories of any kind. Possibly the name "ROUMA" (which is amour (love) spelled backward). You now have someone to confide in... someone who is non-judgmental and with whom you can share your innermost thoughts.

By building this deeply personal and private relationship with your superconscious mind, you will find that you are never alone anymore. You can completely trust in its knowledge and know that it has no ulterior motive - only your best interests at heart - because you are one. It will communicate with you through your intuition and advise you in every decision.

You will no longer have to worry and become distraught, analyzing endlessly every possibility when forced to make decisions. Now you can just LET GO and know your superconscious mind and your inner GOD are always there for you. Trust them, surrender to their profound knowing and truth. You will find the ultimate intimacy.

You have been receiving signals, or messages, from your superconscious mind since birth, but have not understood their origin. When you are not living in proper alignment with your whole self, or when you are in a situation that is not beneficial to your spiritual growth, you will experience any number of the following: your emotions begin to rule, discomfort and disease (dis-ease) are manifested, you may experience a lack of energy, weight problems, accidents, addiction to alcohol, drugs (prescription or otherwise), your sleep patterns may become disturbed (too much, not enough, or interrupted sleep), your appetite may become erratic, etc... All the while, you are looking outside yourself for answers. Instead, accept the message you are receiving and ask ROUMA to point out what it is trying to convey to you. In this way, you will find you are free from the pain of analysis and worry and you will have a feeling of peace and harmony.

GOD created you in his own image, which is perfection. Whenever something happens to you that is not in alignment with this law of perfection, your inner GOD, or superconscious mind, will give you a signal to indicate that you are not on the right path. You are going against the flow. GOD gave us free will so that we would be free to choose our life experiences. Without our trust in his guidance, we will take more time achieving our goals. GOD loves you like a son. Often, parents resist when a son wants to leave home and experience life on his own. They want to protect him - but that attitude will keep him from growing and learning. When parents truly love a child, they trust in him and are there to guide him, but not to live his life for him.

As GOD'S children, we are loved unconditionally and given the freedom to learn our own lessons. HE is always there for us, to guide us and to give us strength and support. HE will always share his wisdom with us, if we ask HIM. All you need to do to master your life is to listen to the messages and to take action.

CHAPTER 2 EXERCISES

» Take a sheet of paper and write down everything you can think of that you now know has been the result of listening to the messages from your subconscious mind. Try to remember as many experiences as you can, pleasant or unpleasant. Perhaps you were afraid something was going to happen and it did. Perhaps you were wishing for something and were surprised when you got it. Without realizing it, you were programming your subconscious mind. As you recall each incident and become conscious of how you made it happen, write it down. You will begin to understand that you have always had the power to design your own life.

» Visualize something specific that you would like to see happen in your life in the near future - over the next few days, perhaps. Keep it simple, but make sure it is of some significance to you and then ask that it happen very soon. Over the few days, think often about it- feel that you have actually attained it. Believe that you are touching it or experiencing it so that you know, firsthand how it feels. Make it seem as real as you possibly can and know deep in your heart that it is coming soon.

» REMEMBER that the subconscious mind understands neither the past nor the future. It only understands the pictures in the HERE AND NOW. So that,when you are doing the second exercise, tell yourself "I am", or "I have". You must be able to clearly see your-self with your result and feel your happiness inside.

» It is important that you keep this exercise to yourself, as to share this with others will dilute the possibility of success. Uncon-sciously, you could be influenced by their doubts and opinions and your subconscious mind will pick it up. Focus clearly on the task at hand.

» Repeat the following affirmation whenever you are alone with your thoughts. You will find that you have finally met your closest friend.

I NOW CONSIDER MY BODY TO BE MY BEST FRIEND AND GUIDE ON EARTH AND I AM RE-LEARNING TO RESPECT, ACCEPT AND LOVE IT AS IT WAS INTENDED.

CHAPTER 3

COMMITMENT & RESPONSIBILITY

RESPONSIBILITY is defined as "a moral obligation to assume the consequences of our choices". EACH OF US IS FUNDAMENTALLY RESPONSIBLE FOR HIS/HER OWN EVOLUTION: thereby each of us is responsible for the outcome of our own "soul purpose". Thus, only we are accountable for our own decisions and must accept the consequences of our actions and reactions. "Human Responsibility" does not mean that we are being held accountable for the decisions of others.

It may be a difficult notion to accept, but you have been responsible for your life since before you were born! You chose your parents, your family life and even the country in which you were born. As long as you have the slightest doubt about this, you will not be in a position to change your life. You must understand this concept and take full responsibility in order to become empowered enough to take control of your life.

If you are unhappy with the consequences of your decisions, change your decisions. ONLY YOU CAN CREATE YOUR LIFE! In understanding this fully, you will also understand that others are also solely responsible for theirs. Let them take on that responsibility for their own sake and yours.

The most precious gift parents can give to their children is self-responsibility. For example: a child decides not to go to school one day because he "doesn't feel like it" and he asks his mother to write a note to his teacher stating that he is sick. What he is doing is making a decision without wanting to assume the consequences. In this case, the mother should write a note stating "My son does not feel like going to school today.", and tell the child: "You have made the decision not to go to school today - I will not lie for you. If you don't want to go to school, that is your decision, but be prepared to face the consequences."

A younger child may test his wings in other ways, for example: on a cold day, he wants to play outside without a jacket. The mother, knowing how cold it is, suggests that he dress warmly. The child refuses. It is unnecessary (and usually ineffective) to press the child any further. If she tells him he will "catch cold out there", he probably will, but if she accepts that it is her child's responsibility to live by his own decisions, she will tell him: "If you should feel cold, come back and get your jacket". The child's attitude will become completely different if he is handed the responsibility of making his own decisions. He will not catch a cold because he has not been programmed to do so - he is not thinking about catching a cold. However, as soon as he realizes that it is colder outside than he thought, he will simply come in and put on his jacket. It is our nature to make our own decisions and children constantly assert their right to do so. If a parent is constantly making his child's decisions, the child will tend to do the opposite of whatever he is told.

How many parents feel they have failed in their parenting? Why? Their children have not met their expectations- they have quit school or become thieves, they've spent time in jail or become drug addicts, or gotten themselves in any number of predicaments. Parents who blame themselves have assumed they are responsible for the decisions and choices made by their children. This is contrary to one of the great natural laws.

Great universal laws have been eternally in place to manage the universe: they are the physical, cosmic, psychic and spiritual laws that will be maintained regardless of how we choose to behave. We will suffer the consequences of contradicting these laws by experiencing disease, accidents and unhappiness. Breaking physical laws results in very obvious consequences. For example, a person drinking a glass of poison because "it looks like water, so it can't be bad", finds out that his body will react violently. He has broken a physical law. Believing or not in a particular truth does not alter the truth.

The Law of Responsibility is part of the Law of Love, touching the depths of the soul. We are each responsible for ourselves - our "being", our "belongings". Feeling responsible for the actions and feelings of others can result in our own feelings of guilt. This is very uncomfortable for us, even more so when the expectations we have toward others are unmet. Disappointment, anger and frustration are the result - all of which cause despair and disease.

Every situation you encounter in your life is an opportunity for growth and personal evolution. Having chosen your own parents and your children, you have intentionally brought specific lessons forward to be learned in your life. Failure to acknowledge or take responsibility that you have chosen those around you for a reason will cause a great deal of unpleasantness because you will not understand why "negative" things are happening to you in regard to them.

As a parent, the most important lesson you can teach your children, as early as possible, is that they are self-responsible. If your 16-year old wants to quit school because he feels he is not learning anything of any value, I suggest you say to him: "The decision is yours, son, but consider the consequences. Do you realize that you will limit your choice of jobs and your income without a diploma? You will likely never do what you would really enjoy for a living without the proper education. Are you comfortable with that?" If he answers in the affirmative and he has made this decision on his own (without peer pressure), it is better to let him live out his own life experience. If you do not, he will do whatever it takes to challenge you and make you react. Remember, he can always go back to school.

If you are a parent or plan on becoming one, I'm sure the prospect of handing personal responsibility over to your children is unsettling. You are convinced you are responsible for them. Be assured, your only responsibility as a parent is to love and guide your children. Remember your own childhood - what stands out in your mind as being of primary importance? Not this or that toy, but the love and support of your parents. The most critical element in the child/parent relationship, or in any other relationship for that matter, is love. I will define love's true meaning in Chapter 4.

COMMITMENT is automatically implied when deciding to have a child. In entering a relationship of any kind, commitment is a "given". I will explain this fully.

You are not responsible for the happiness of the people around you, whether they are friends, family or co-workers. WHAT YOU ARE RESPONSIBLE FOR IS THE WAY YOU REACT TOWARD THE ATTITUDE PEOPLE HAVE TOWARD YOU. It is said that "You do not judge the worth of a man by what others say about him, but by what he says about others." When others are gentle, violent, critical or loving toward you, it is because you made it happen. Others are your mirror. The way they react toward you is based on the way you react toward yourself unconsciously. You must learn from this.

For example: If a certain person is very disagreeable and critical around you and you judge him as a disagreeable and critical person, it is because the you are disagreeable and critical with yourself and this person, being your mirror, is only there to help you become conscious of this. If you accept the fact that you are this way, I mean really accept, you will not be bothered by or attract disagreeable or critical people anymore.

A change in your own attitude will give you the impression that others around you are changing. The fact is, there is good in everyone - it is up to you to see it. Your thinking is all you have control of - you cannot control others, but your perception of them will change.

You are beginning to understand the notion of personal RESPONSIBILITY! That is why it is so important to become conscious of who you are inwardly - so that you can change your perception and, ultimately your reality.

COMMITMENT is defined as a pledge of one's self to a position or a course of action. Commitments can be verbal or written, as in a contract, which binds you to another, whether it be an employee, a spouse, a partner, etc.

Parents make a commitment to their children when they decide to bring them into the world. That commitment entails providing the basic needs of life i.e.: food, shelter, education, love, respect and guidance. It does not mean that they must provide everything material that the children desire. The extras are not part of the basic commitment.

In a work situation, an employee is committed to fulfilling his job responsibilities and his employer is committed to paying him and to providing a safe and efficient work environment.

When one makes a commitment at home, at work or otherwise, even by agreeing to meet someone at a certain time for an appointment or whatever, it is important on a soul level to keep the commitment. "YOU REAP WHAT YOU SOW" is one of the greatest laws of life - your integrity and your word are vital to your overall being. You cannot disengage yourself from responsibility, but you can disengage yourself from a previous commitment. Before doing so, be sure to evaluate the consequences, as it can be the precursor to problems in relationships. Before making such decisions, always ask yourself "What will this cost me in regard to my relationships, health, happiness, love...?" Remember - you always reap what you sow.

Here's an example: Perhaps you had promised to meet someone for a social engagement, but something came up in the meantime that you would prefer to do. You have a dilemma, you risk the other person feeling hurt by canceling your plans and pleasing yourself, or you (once again) find yourself spending the evening doing something you'd rather not be doing, pleasing others instead of yourself and possibly resenting them and yourself for it. The best solution is to call the person to whom you've made the commitment and be honest with them. Tell them something has come up that you really don't want to miss and work out a compromise. If you are sincere and straightforward, he will respect you for it.

The same applies in your relationship with yourself. If, for example, you've promised yourself you will exercise every morning.

You have made a commitment to yourself. You adhere strictly to your exercise routine for the first few days, but gradually you begin to neglect your commitment. You can't find the time...you forget...finally the inevitable happens; you have completely stopped exercising. Instead of feeling guilty or becoming critical of yourself, treat yourself as you would a dear friend. Remind yourself that there is no need to be so hard on yourself - accept that you may not have been quite ready to make that commitment for whatever reason and try again to do so when you feel more prepared. Remind yourself that you have a responsibility to yourself and to those you love to be the best you can be - that you owe it to yourself and to them to be healthy. When you fully understand your reasons for making the commitment to exercise in the first place, you will be ready to do so. Detach yourself from the situation long enough to become objective about it instead of instilling guilt and anger in yourself. Before you know it, you will be happily exercising on a regular basis because you are ready to and have made it a very positive experience.

In relationships where you find yourself living with other people, it is essential that each member of the household understand that they have a commitment to the other members to carry their own weight. In a communal situation, everyone must contribute to the care and upkeep of the home. I would suggest that regular family meetings be established to determine the distribution of household chores and to evaluate on a regular basis how these chores are being carried out. Open discussion regarding the running of the home will ensure harmony and order. This applies whether the occupants are family, a couple, room-mates or bunk-mates.

Children will learn a great deal from these negotiations, about what it takes to actually run a home, how to interact with others in a team situation, and how to deal with consequences. This method applies whether you are living with a family, sharing with other singles, or living as a couple. WE CAN HAVE EXPECTATIONS ONLY WHEN CLEAR COMMITMENTS HAVE BEEN MADE.

Tell yourself "I will do", not "I will try". A clear commitment indicates certainty of action. Otherwise, there will be misunderstanding and disharmony.

CHAPTER 3 EXERCISES

» Choose a current situation in which you feel someone else is responsible for what is happening to you. Determine your own responsibility regarding the situation, and write it down. What commitments have you made regarding your responsibilities? Now get in touch with that person and go over, in detail, what is expected of each of you until it is clear to you and to the other.

» Is there a current situation in which you feel responsible for someone else? Accept that that person is ultimately responsible for their own life, their choices and their decisions. Now, contact this person and discuss the issue of personal commitment until clear commitments have been determined.

» Take a sheet of paper and list all the promises and commitments you can think of that you have made to yourself and to others. Which ones have you kept? Are there some from which you can comfortably disengage yourself? From this exercise, you will realize that there are many instances in which you have made commitments that you cannot possibly keep or that you would really prefer not to keep.

» Write down what you need or want to commit to at this point in your life, both for yourself and for others. Be fair to them and to yourself and be conscious of whether you are overextending yourself. Be conscious, also, of your intent in each situation, remembering that you are not responsible for the happiness of others. Again, contact each of the people involved and make the responsibilities of each of these commitments clear to them and to yourself.

» Repeat the following affirmation every moment you can, until you understand it fully. Then go on to the next chapter.

I AM THE ONLY PERSON RESPONSIBLE FOR MY LIFE AND I ALLOW EVERYONE AROUND ME TO BE RESPONSIBLE FOR THEIRS.

CHAPTER 4

LOVE AND POSSESSION

LOVE! What a wonderful word! I have worked with thousands of people over the past 25 years and they all assured me they knew how to love - it was everyone else who was getting it wrong!

If you are like most people, you will say "I love my mate, my children, my parents, etc. but I feel my relationships are not what I would like them to be. Somehow I am dissatisfied." Most of you are realizing that the dissatisfaction has been there for much too long. There must be something more - something better somewhere.

WHAT IS LOVE?

Love is giving someone all the space and freedom they need. It is also respecting our own needs for space and freedom. Love is respecting and accepting what other people wish to accomplish in their lives. Love is learning to respect and and accept others opinions even though we may not agree with or understand them. Love is also giving and guiding without any expectations.

Make it your life's goal RIGHT NOW to learn to love with your whole heart. Most people understand the kind of love that comes from the mind: the one that gives you permission to run other people's lives, the one that makes you want to change people and tell them what to do. Even though your intentions may be good and you are convinced your "assistance" is in their best interest, what you are exhibiting is not love, it is POSSESSIVE LOVE. What goes on in other peoples lives are their business, not yours. Free yourself to love unconditionally and others will respond in the same way.

We continuously judge and analyze the behavior of others because we have expectations from them. Again, love is giving and guiding without any expectations. Learn to love in this way.

Here is an example of loving with the mind: A woman's husband came home one evening and told her that he had decided to have a garden for the summer. Here's how the conversation went:

"Darling, I feel like having a garden this summer."

"Why? That doesn't make any sense! You never get home from work till after 9 p.m. - you'll never find the time!"

"I really feel like having a garden - if I find I don't have the time to look after it properly, I'm sure our son will help me."

"You should know that son of ours by now (18 years old) - what makes you think he would bother with your garden!? You're just going to make more work for yourself."

After further discussion, he finally gave in and changed his mind about the garden. The rest of the evening, the woman felt somehow disturbed. Her husband sat glued to the television set and remained silent. She found herself eating out of frustration. She knew she had forced her views on him and that somehow that was inappropriate, but she had believed it was really in his best interest. Why did she feel so bad?

Deep down, this woman loves her husband and was only trying to prevent him from overextending himself, but she was loving him with her mind and not with her heart. Had she been loving from her heart, she should have said "If it makes you happy, darling, have your garden". If the garden went to seed, what difference would it have made in her life? Perhaps a garden was just the excuse her husband needed to come home from work a little earlier - it could only have been a positive experience for him. If the garden were to become neglected, he at least would have had the satisfaction of doing what pleased him for awhile.

You see, TO LOVE is to accept and respect the other person's wishes, whether or not we understand or agree with them.

I could quote many such examples, but all that is needed is to understand that loving entails respect of others' needs, wants and of their space. Whenever we try to control someone else's words or thoughts, we are not respecting their space. In doing so, you are also losing your own space. With both of your spaces being intermingled in this manner, each of you is suffocating the other.

Every living thing needs its space - its room to grow. Crowding a number of trees into a space that is meant for one will stunt the growth of all the trees. It works the same way with human beings. Our individual space is vital. Some of us need a little more space than others. Children and adults who are strong-willed and independent need more space than most other people.

You will find as you begin to grow spiritually, that you will require more space. From this space, you can maintain your balance and reach out to others with strength and clarity. That is why children can love unconditionally; their space has not been cluttered by others. Observe and learn from the children around you.

In loving someone fully and unconditionally, you may not always agree with that person, but you will accept them without trying to change them. It is the ego that assumes your way of thinking is the correct one. It is the ego that builds expectations.

Naturally, we would like those we love to be happy - but we base that on our notion of happiness. If your son decides to take drugs, it is because he needs to experience something through drugs. It is not up to you, as a parent, or up to anyone else to judge , to ridicule or to try to control his life. The responsibility of his decision is his. He will stop when he has learned what he needs to learn and he will have to face the consequences on his own. No one can do it for him. Although it is difficult to stand back and watch, feeling helpless, it is more dangerous for that child to be surrounded by parents who tell him that he is wrong and do everything to try and stop him. He will only react by using more drugs in order to challenge their authority.

Guide him lovingly and point out the consequences without judging him. Tell him: "Listen, I don't agree with what you're doing and I am afraid for you but if that is what you think you need to do, I will respect your decision. When you decide you want to talk about it, I'll be here for you". Give him his space. He will respect you and will learn to respect himself once he has learned to take responsibility for his actions. Let him know that you respect him by telling him that you are confident he is capable of making the right decision. When he decides he needs help, he will have enough trust and confidence in your relationship to ask you for it.

Love and respect go hand-in-hand. Respect other people's individuality, including your children's. If your children want to wear their hair long, not to study, or to eat and think differently, it is their choice. It is part of who they are right now. Show your children this way of loving as early on as possible. Be sure they understand, even as babies, that their parents will respect and guide them always and that they will be responsible and accountable for their own decisions. Ensure that they are safe and give them their space. Those children will evolve quickly and be better prepared to manage their own lives.

We make decisions as best we can based on the knowledge we have at the time. That is why it's so important to accept our decisions and not waste time regretting them. That's also why it's important to accept the decisions of others. They are making the best possible decisions at the time. If someone you love makes a decision you disagree with or you feel is inappropriate, share your knowledge with them, but not your opinion. Tell them: "If that is what makes you happy, go ahead"...and mean it. Can you imagine what that sentence can do to a relationship? How would you have liked hearing that when you were a child? How wonderful it would have been had your parents had such faith and confidence in you!

If a young child is merely testing you by telling you they are going to do something that you think is utterly ridiculous, say: "If that is what really makes you happy, go ahead"...and mean it. Rest assured that they will think twice before doing it when the decision to do so is actually theirs. Their common sense will kick in much earlier if you leave them to their own devices.

I must caution you though, that understanding the notion of "space" in this context, is very important. When allowing others to go ahead with their plans, make sure they do not trespass on your space.

If a friend were to say: "I thought it would be nice if we could go to a movie together tonight" when you already had other plans, you are under no obligation to go unless you want to and you should feel free to say "I'm sorry, I have other plans or, I don't feel like going tonight." It's that simple. In no way are you responsible for your friend's happiness. If, however, you would like to go to the movie and need to cancel other plans to do so, feel free to cancel them considerately and fairly. Whatever you do, do it without any expectations and ask yourself if it will make you happy. Try not to step on other peoples' toes whenever possible, but always keep in mind that your own happiness is your primary responsibility. This is not selfish. You did not come to this earth to make sure everyone else is happy. You will begin to realize that you (and everyone else) is only disappointed when their expectations have not been met.

Here's another example: A husband, having had a wonderful day, decides he will treat his wife to a special evening out. Rather than calling to ask her if she would like to go, he phones and says: "Darling, I feel terrific tonight! I had a super day at work and have decided to take you out. Get ready! I will pick you up and we'll go to a fancy restaurant". The evening goes well enough - they have a nice time, but something is missing in it for her. She never took the time to ask herself if that's what she really wanted to do that particular night. She "went along with it" unconsciously, just to please him. She was not in the same frame of mind that he was in. When they return home, he expects her to make love to him...but she doesn't feel like it. He is disappointed because his expectations have not been met. Had they both been conscious of what the other was feeling during the evening, it may have ended on a much more pleasant note.

This is how the scenario may have been played out, had the husband been loving from his heart and not taken his partner for granted: "Darling, I feel terrific tonight! I had a super day and I feel like celebrating with you. Would you join me for a beautiful dinner and we could celebrate together?" He would have no expectations because, with this frame of mind, he is not "taking her out", rather, she is joining him in sharing the celebration". The difference seems subtle but the results will be worlds apart! Clear communication avoids a great deal of misunderstanding.

We should never take anything for granted. the decision is not ours to make, always check with the other person involved. This is a very important part in loving and respecting others.

Most of the problems in relationships between husbands and wives, parents and children - even in the workplace - stem from expectations and poor communication. Because we are not conscious of our actions and thoughts most of the time, our relationships tend to remain on the level of possession and manipulation. Accept and understand that no one is responsible for anyone else's happiness! When someone wants to please you or you want to please them, it is icing on the cake! LEARN TO BAKE YOUR OWN CAKE - ENJOY IT ON YOUR OWN! If someone wants to enjoy your cake with you, to share your happiness -THAT'S ICING ON THE CAKE!

Think about your mate for a moment. Are there things you would like to change about him/her? Remember that you chose your particular mate because you had something to learn from him/her (life lessons). If you were to leave the relationship before completing your lessons or refuse to learn them even after the separation, you will find yourself in another relationship with the same problems...maybe worse! Wouldn't it be wiser to learn to love your mate unconditionally and to accept his/her choice of being? You'll be surprised how much happier you both will be and how quickly your relationship will improve.

If a separation becomes necessary for each of you to grow, it should be harmonious. Both partners must be convinced that it is the best choice for them. When there is a disagreeable separation and the couple parts on angry terms, they are only trying to escape from a situation in which they could not accept or tolerate each other. We can't run and we can't hide. As long as we refuse to learn how to love each other properly, the situation will reoccur indefinitely. Considering how uncomfortable that is, wouldn't it be easier to learn to love right now?

Here is another example of someone who believes she loves with her heart, but proves she is loving with her mind, thus creating expectations and the resulting disappointment:

A woman has a dear friend who is having a birthday party. She spends a great deal of time finding them "just the right gift" - something she would really have like to receive herself. When they receive it, they do not react the way she had hoped. She is disappointed and frustrated and a little angry inside. She spent a lot of time and money to get them "just the right gift" and they didn't appreciate it. That's loving with the mind.

When loving from the heart, the scenario would be played out more like this:

"I feel like buying you a gift for your birthday - what would make you happy?" (You may mention monetary restrictions, where applicable).

Ask him for a few ideas or suggestions. This way, neither of you will be disappointed! Perhaps he would honestly prefer not to receive a gift and says: "I would like you to share in celebrating my birthday, but would prefer no gifts". Respect that, if it is meant sincerely. If, deep down, he would like a gift and can't bring himself to say so, he will soon learn to be open and honest about his wishes.

On the other hand, if you enjoy surprising someone with a special gift, understand that you may be doing so, at least in part, to please yourself. It gives you pleasure to shop for the gift, to wrap it and to anticipate the response. If you are honest about receiving pleasure from the process, you will enjoy it even more - even if the gift is not well-received. Be sure, when presenting a gift, to mention that you have kept the receipt and that, if the gift is unsuitable for any reason, the recipient is free to exchange it with no expectations and no hard feelings on your part.

When someone decides to discuss a project with you that they have in mind, they have already thought it through. Accept their ideas as they present them and offer your opinion only if it is asked for. If you really can't hold back, ask their permission first by saying "Would you mind if I gave you my opinion on this?" Otherwise, an unwanted opinion is often perceived as a judgment and is usually unwelcome. Simply, it is none of your concern.

It becomes your concern only when the decisions of others affect your space. If, for example, you are the parent of a teenage son who decides that what makes him happy is to have his friends visit at two o'clock in the morning and to play loud music that would affect your space. You would then have the right to assert yourself by saying "I'm sorry, but at this hour, I need to sleep. This house belongs to everyone and we must respect one another". Be sure to explain that he is welcome to play his loud music when you are not at home.

On the other hand, if he chooses to come home very late at night when you would prefer an earlier curfew, you create useless expectations. As long as he does not wake you, the choice is his what hour he comes home. He will pay the consequences of losing too much sleep and will have learned to make a more appropriate decision in the future. It will not affect your life if he is tired the next day, but arguing with him about curfew will definitely cause discord in your relationship. Trust him and respect him enough to know that he will make the right choices and remember that the road to success is not perfectly straight. He will spend several tired days before he learns how to find the right balance for himself.

Why waste energy and complicate your life worrying about someone else's hairstyle, clothing or "weird" ideas...or whether or not they share your notion of happiness? LIVE AND LET LIVE! We waste so much energy worrying about other people's business that we don't have the energy to take care of our own.

It is often stated that "YOU CAN'T LOVE OTHERS UNTIL YOU'VE LEARNED TO LOVE YOURSELF". Few people really understand what this means. In truly loving yourself or others, the two essential ingredients are RESPECT and ACCEPTANCE. Your relationships with others will improve a thousand-fold once you have learned to love and respect yourself. Respect your own space and you will be able to respect the space of others. Accept yourself as you are and grow from there and you will learn to accept others as they are. Your relationships will flourish.

Treat yourself firmly but gently - do not judge yourself when you have done something that you think is non-beneficial to you (some would call this a 'mistake'...but it is actually a 'learning experi-ence'). Often this is the only way to become acquainted with a par-ticular "consequence". Continue to learn and grow, maintaining your own garden (your inner self), your own space, and everything around you will begin to exhibit balance and harmony.

Find peace in your garden and there will be no place for guilt. (Guilt will be discussed further in another chapter.)

As you reap what you sow, doesn't it make sense to sow as much love as you can? You will probably answer: "But why should I do all the work?" Loving others is not work, it is a blessing. You feel that you could be nicer to other people if they were only nicer to you. That would be like saying: "If they would only plant some carrots, I would be in a position to eat some!" Start planting! YOU WILL REAP WHAT YOU SOW!

Love has tremendous healing power. It is a powerful vibration. When you are filled with love, those vibrations are so strong that people around you will feel better in your presence. You will think that others have changed, but they are only responding to your posi-tive vibration. Again, they are your mirror.

What does it mean to "LET GO"? How does it happen? It hap-pens when you decide to stop wanting to change others or yourself. It happens when you just accept yourself and others as they are, unconditionally...and when it happens, the transformation begins. You will begin to witness miracles!

The more you practice unconditional love, the more you have small victories, the easier it becomes and your happiness and fulfillment will accelerate. Never forget that when you judge or criticize others, you are implying that you are superior. This is not so. Nobody is better than anybody else. Everyone, even the most hardened criminal is born to love and be loved. THERE ARE NO BAD PEOPLE, ONLY SUFFERING PEOPLE.

By accepting suffering, whether it be your own or someone else's, it is much easier to accept violence, even if you do not agree with it. Once you understand the suffering of a criminal, you will realize that, because we all reap what we sow, they are learning their life's lessons also. They are suffering inside and are inflicting suffering onto others. When they feel acceptance, they will feel loved. Only then will they understand suffering and be transformed. They will no longer be able to inflict it onto others.

By sowing love, you will automatically reap love. Like learning to dance, the more you practice and the more you discipline yourself, the more you will succeed and the happier you will be.

CHAPTER 4 EXERCISES

» Think of one simple thing that would bring you happiness and do it.

» Ask one other person what simple thing would bring them happiness and help them accomplish it. If it requires an investment of time and/or money on your part, be sure to discuss your limitations.

» In summary, take the time to consciously bring yourself one piece of happiness at a time and to do the same for someone else.

» Repeat the following affirmation every moment you can until you understand it fully. Then go on to the next chapter.

I RESPECT AND ACCEPT THE WISHES AND OPINIONS OF OTHERS WHETHER OR NOT I AGREE WITH OR UNDERSTAND THEIR REASONS. CONSEQUENTLY, I RADIATE AND RECEIVE MORE AND MORE LOVE.

CHAPTER 5

CAUSE AND EFFECT

Understanding the immutable Cosmic Law of Cause and Effect will help you become the master of your own destiny. Simply put, action causes reaction or "you reap what you sow". What you put into your life is what you will get out of it.

Cause and Effect is a Universal Law governing the physical, mental, psychic, cosmic and spiritual worlds. Not to "believe in it" is just as senseless as denying the law of gravity. While telling yourself there is no such thing as gravity, jump off the top of your desk and notice how long you will stay in the air. The Law of Gravity exists. While planting beans, tell yourself that you will be harvesting carrots. What do you think you will be harvesting? Exactly. You reap what you sow, just as you do in life. Everything you reap in your life was sown in your conscious and unconscious thoughts. Those are the seeds of your reality, so be aware of what you are planting.

I could cite thousands of examples relating to this law. Here are only a few:

Right now, do you think it is possible for you to be living in a million dollar house? No? It's not for you - it's only for "rich people", right? There you are! You reap according to your thoughts. Why is it there are so many people living in mansions? There are thousands of millionaires! Why them and not you? Only because THEY BELIEVE IN IT!

Would you like to take a vacation for a whole year? You answer: "I can't do that - I'd sure like to, but it's impossible - no money, no time - where would I go?!" So you stay.

Do you believe illnesses are hereditary? I see. You probably think you have no choice in the matter. You will never have any other option as long as you don't believe you do. You will create this

47

in your life because you believe it to be so. You have accepted the idea that diseases are hereditary and that is your truth. Did you know that scientists are discovering that there are fewer and fewer "hereditary" diseases? Although there may be genetic predispositions to disease, the only "hereditary" disease I acknowledge is the way of thinking that is transmitted from generation to generation.

The Law of Cause and Effect is there for all of us, just like gravity. It singles out no race, no gender, no economic or social position. Whether you are rich or poor, Pope or beggar, man, woman or child, this law exists for you. Every time you attempt to ignore this law, you will suffer the consequences. To be able to determine the effect of any particular cause can often require great wisdom.

If your life is spent in laziness, waiting for rewards to be presented to you on a silver platter, you will never acquire the same degree of success as someone who expresses good will and works diligently. Many people are constantly envying others, watching others' successes, believing they will never get the chance themselves. They will reap what they've sown and that is that.

If you feel there is not enough love in your life, who forgot to sow some? If there is not enough affection being shown to you, who forgot to sow some? Showing affection insincerely or with expectations will not result in a rich harvest of affection. Expectations come from the mind, not from the heart. Show love and affection from the heart, without expectations and enjoy the harvest! You cannot reap from someone else's heart if you remain in your mind. "A heart-to-heart talk" is certainly much different from a "chat" or a "conversation", is it not? It is open, sincere, without boundaries or barriers. Love that way, heart-to-heart.

If you want to change the effects and the results in any area of your life, you only have to change their causes. Take a look at what you reap and look back to verify what you have sown. Undoubtedly, you will find the cause.

Sit too close to a fire and you will get burned. Touch an ice cube with your bare hands and they will get cold. Too simple? The Law of

Cause and Effect is no more complicated than that when applied to every area of your life.

Reaction is in accordance to action. Humans specialize in complicating their lives when dealing with such simple principles. They become helplessly confused by worrying, doubting and by being afraid. They end up nowhere. Take a moment to look inside yourself before you determine the direction you will go. Is it really where you want to end up?

If you don't understand why some situations keep repeating themselves in your life, remember that what you reap has been sown by you from as far back as your childhood. If you decided as a young child to feel sorry for yourself, you will continue to do so into adulthood. This particular programming may manifest itself as poor health, emotional illness or a violent temper. You probably do not remember making such decisions, because they are usually made unconsciously.

However, it is not necessary to go as far back as your early childhood in order to understand the concept. You can start a new chapter of your life RIGHT NOW! You can change the effects you are experiencing by starting this minute to change the causes. If you decide that, starting this minute, you want to reap more love in your life, start sowing it everywhere. It grows very quickly and can be harvested and enjoyed even when newly sprouted. Stop wasting any more time worrying about the past! All there is, is NOW - make it work for you - it's right there for you to use!

Sow what you want to reap! Start thinking abundance, if that's what you desire. If you enjoy a fancy restaurant instead of a cafeteria, go there! Enjoy it - live according to your true nature and your subconscious mind will quickly reprogram itself to manifest exactly who you are, but be certain it is who you really are. Be true to yourself and change your attitude accordingly. Think and say only words that you want to be the seeds of what you sow. If you believe that by eating in a fancy restaurant you will be unable to pay your rent, that's exactly what will happen. You must constantly program yourself in accordance with your goals! Tell yourself "I am rich, I experience abundance everywhere. I may not know where it comes from, but I believe in my heart that I am provided for by a Great Universal Source. Abundance is there for me!"

Don't go to extremes or beyond your reasonable limits. Start with small achievements, knowing precisely what your goals are. Are you ready to take action?

You must take action in order to get the desired reaction, or result. Sitting at home and thinking about it is not going to get you results. Clarify your goal and put your energy into achieving it - only then will you move forward.

If you want a new wardrobe, get rid of your old clothes that you don't wear anymore. Pretend you are merely making room in your closet for all the new clothes you have just purchased so that you are able to clearly visualize them in the closet. Then, as you purchase them, piece by piece, put your new clothes in their place.

You're probably telling yourself: "Sure - it can't be that simple. If it were that simple I would have done it long ago. There's no way it's possible." Do you see the cause you are putting in motion? Be conscious of each one of your thoughts. What were you thinking about when you read those lines? Do you believe in them? Are you still doubting the whole process or are you ready to get started? Doubting will get you nowhere. Take action. You have nothing to lose and everything to gain.

If you want to be surrounded by friends and have an active life, start acting that way. Find new friends; go where there are other people -start conversations wherever you go and do it every day. You will put a new cause into motion by taking action.

Here are the basic steps to getting what you want:

– Clearly determine what you want and visualize it.
– Live it in your mind until you can touch it, taste it and deeply feel the joy in it.
– Take action.

REMEMBER: YOU WILL ONLY GET WHAT YOU EXPECT TO RECEIVE!

The rewards may not come instantly, but DON'T GIVE UP! Perseverance is essential.

Once you fully understand the Law of Cause and Effect you will realize that it is foolish to take revenge on anyone. If you feel someone has caused you pain, it is not your place to punish them in any way. By letting go, you will no longer feel a need to judge or punish others. Most of the time, the other person never meant to cause you any pain. It is only the way that you perceived it that hurt you. If someone said or did something and they only wanted to help you but you perceived it in a negative way, they will not reap anything other than their intentions. Just because you perceive something to be wrong does not make it so. You can only see things through your beliefs. Always try and see what the other persons' intentions were, that way you will most likely not get upset as much as before. When you hold a grudge, you stop talking to someone, you sulk and get angry, say harsh words and make demands that others change themselves to meet your expectations... this kind of behavior indicates that you believe you are superior to others; that you are GOD and that they are something much less. You are saying to them "I will show you how to be perfect, like I am". Stop wasting your energy.

Like I said, if you feel someone has hurt you, it is not your place to punish them in any way. The Law of Cause and Effect will take care of the situation in accordance with the <u>intent</u> of the other person toward you. He will reap what he has sown. It is in your best interest in terms of your own health and well-being to detach yourself from the situation and to accept people as they are. They have not hurt you - you have allowed yourself to feel hurt. Revenge would have a negative impact on you in terms of your own spiritual growth. You will reap something negative because your intentions were negative. It is important to get past any such feelings.

CHAPTER 5 EXERCISES

» Make a list of the goals you would like to reach by tomorrow. Do the same for the goals you would like to reach over the next week and the next year. The only limitations are those that you will place on yourself.

» Over the next three days, become more conscious of the negative and unnecessary attitudes that could become obstacles in your achieving these goals. Transform these thoughts into positive ones that will help you get what you want. Take a close look at your attitude!

» Repeat the following affirmation as often as you can. Go on to the next chapter.

AS OF NOW I SOW AND I REAP WITH MY THOUGHTS, WORDS AND ACTIONS, ONLY WHAT IS BENEFICIAL TO ME.

CHAPTER 6

THE TIES THAT BIND

The "ties" that I refer to are the invisible cords that have been forming since your birth - the ones that , because of your reactions, continue to bind you to those who have been authority figures in your life; parents, grandparents, older siblings, relatives, baby-sitters, neighbors, teachers, etc. Whatever you refused to accept in them produced a lingering bond that continues to keep you tied to those people and situations.

Try to recall your early childhood from birth to seven years old and think of those who were close enough to you to have an impact on your very being. Babies and young children live by their instincts and accept what they experience and what they are told as fact. Although instinct prevails, they are making conscious decisions about what goes on around them.

The first decision you ever made in this life, although you will not remember, was choosing your parents. In choosing them, you were accepting and loving them as they were. Even so, right from birth, you would surely have liked to change some of their behavior as it pertained to you. Each attitude not accepted has formed a "cord". This invisible tie, always present between you and your parents, creates an inner irritation. It remains there to remind you that you are exactly like what you did not like in your parents. This is true of everyone you have ever judged.

Here are some examples: Perhaps your father was a withdrawn person. He kept his thoughts to himself, never expressed his feelings or communicated with others. You rarely spoke with him and he never told you he loved you. By not accepting the way he was, you felt very frustrated. Take a look at your own behavior now. Are you open with other people, expressing your thoughts and feelings honestly - or do you say what others want to hear? If you did not accept your father's behavior, you probably will find yourself exhibiting the same behavior.

Was your mother overbearing, overprotective, always encroaching on your space? Was she always giving you unwanted advice and telling you how to live your life? If you found it unbearable, unacceptable, take a look at your own behavior now. If you have any doubt about how others interpret your current behavior, just ask them. They will probably tell you that you are "just like your mother!"

If you refused to accept a parent's authority, you have inherited it now. You may express it differently, but it is there nonetheless.

If you could not accept that one of your parents was submissive, take a good look at your own behavior. Do you do things consistently out of obligation, or because you want to do them?

Was your mother extremely fussy about cleanliness? How do you feel about untidiness and disorder? Probably the same.

Having reviewed these examples, you may find something you did not accept about your mother that you cannot find any trace of in your present attitude.

"I am the opposite!" you will say. You have probably put so much effort into being the opposite of your mother, that you are preventing yourself from expressing your own personality. Whether you are exactly the same or determined to be the opposite, you are still reacting and carrying that baggage with you. In trying so desperately to be different from your mother, the cord is even harder to break than if you were the same.

As long as you continue to react to the behavior of others who influenced you, you will not be free to pursue your own personal goals. Your vision will be constantly blurred by the past and you will repeat the same mistakes over and over again.

Situations involving violence are the most difficult to accept. It is critical to your development that you resolve this in your heart, if you were the victim of any type of violence. If you do not acknowledge and get past your inherent anger about this and your lack of for-giveness, you will discover at the most inopportune time that it has been lying just under the surface, ready to erupt. I'm sure you've worked diligently for many years keeping this all inside of you, but the inner battle will continue unless you consciously break the tie.

Whatever you have failed to let go of in your past has a tendency to resurface over and over again in your present life. Look around you right now at those who occupy your everyday life. Are there things that bother you about their behavior? It bothers you because there is something you need to learn about yourself. Once you ac-knowledge and accept that, it won't bother you any more. BREAK THE TIE AND BREAK THE CYCLE!

Eventually you will learn to love others in spite of indifference, violence, over-protectiveness or rejection because you will learn to see the fears behind their actions. If you felt, for example, that you were the result of an unwanted pregnancy, you may feel a sense of rejection that could carry on throughout your life and in every area of your life. Cut the cord - free yourself to be who you really are and allow yourself to grow. Once you have cut loose, you will evolve quickly and easily.

If you are a parent today, take a look at what your attitude is to-ward your children. Do you find that you are frequently telling them off, reprimanding or punishing them? Do you use harsh words with them? You know that you love them, but you want to make sure they learn your way of doing things - "the right way". You are loving them with your mind and not your heart, just as your parents loved you. When you lose patience with someone, it is only because you are not expressing your love from the heart - only from the head. You are afraid to tell them how you really feel by fear of not being taken seriously. You do not want them repeating the same mistakes you made. That is understandable, but they must live their own lives and learn in their own way.

In order to break this tie with your parents and finally give your-self permission to be who you really are, you must accept that your parents (or other authority figure) did what they could to the best of their knowledge. They loved you the best they knew how and in the only way they knew how.

It may sound odd, but the indifference expressed by truly loving parents is usually synonymous with trust. By loving a child uncon-ditionally, a parent is in tune with the child's essence and abilities. In being so attuned, the parents know that the child is fully capable of making his own decisions. The child knows that the parents will al-ways be there to support them. It is impossible to understand the dy-namics of any relationship from the outside, so do not judge parents who seem indifferent to their children.

Parents who "ride" their children constantly, who are critical and demanding, actually believe that their children are not living up to their potential. These parents are living with unreasonably high ex-pectations - yet there is still love behind each word of criticism.

Other parents will do everything in their power to protect their children from having to face any difficulties or challenges in their lives. Those parents may have had difficult lives themselves and feel they are honestly helping their children by over-protecting them. The reverse is true. It is necessary to the basic growth and maturation of children to learn to make decisions when faced with challenging situations. At the same time, a father who is a weak, submissive man may use violence toward his son to "toughen him up" so that he won't turn out the same way he did. He loves his son, but is loving from his mind. Often, mothers will make tremendous demands on a daughter, "pushing" her into participating and excel-ling at any number of endeavors, to ensure that the daughter has a "better life" than the mother had.

These parents have not severed their own ties with their past and the results are seen in their style of parenting.

Most parents want their children to have more than they did, to become more successful, but this desire often results in unrealistic expectations. Over-protectiveness or excessive strictness toward a child is a manifestation of a very possessive kind of love. THE

MORE ONE FEARS, THE MORE ONE LOVES WITH THE MIND! Please remember the definition of LOVE: *"To love is to accept even if you do not understand or agree."*

There isn't a child on earth who agrees completely with his parents' way of loving because each human being is unique. All children, regardless of cultural background or social status, would have preferred to be loved differently. Each parent has their own way of being and their own lessons to learn. We must accept that our parents were and are still evolving. Put everything that bothered us about their parenting behind us and let go!

The knowledge that there is a love greater than possessive love is relatively recent. Years ago, parents did not have this information and could only love based on what they knew. People in our culture had not acknowledged or understood the existence of inner potential. Happiness was dependent on those around them, so it became imperative that they have some control over the behavior of others. How could your parents teach you a way of loving that they didn't know themselves?

If you add up all the things you wanted to change in your parents and continue to dwell on all the conflict and all the blame , you will see that, over the years, the cord has grown to be quite large. Once you begin to understand that they loved you, in spite of how they expressed it, the best way they knew how, that love was behind every action, every word, you will cut the cord little by little until your heart begins to overflow with love for them. You will see them with new eyes and will know, deep in your heart, how much they really loved you.

Any grudge you hold against someone whose influence has made a lasting impression, holds you prisoner by creating a tie. These ties create an underlying dissatisfaction that affects everything in your life. You are unhappy inside. Now that you know that you can get past this unhappiness by letting go of the hurt and the grudges that you are carrying with you, you will discover an extraordinary freedom. Free your heart to love and to be loved and you'll never look back!

In order to sever these ties, it is not necessary to understand the parent. Only your mind wants to understand, your heart doesn't need to understand, it accepts as is. You only have to feel the love that person had for you at the time. Your heart knows this feeling, not your head. Get past trying to reason. Get in touch with your feelings. In order to forgive these people, you'll naturally find yourself going through the following thought processes, or something similar:

"I know their life was not easy - they had a large family, they were poor. My mother was going through difficult times...etc." Forget all that! Reach in and feel their love - and your love for them. Feel their fears, their weaknesses and their limitations. You may find this frightening, at first, as it may open floodgates of emotion for you. You may have unearthed a love that you had buried many years ago.

Most of us are afraid to accept people as they are. In our mind, it is like saying: "I agree with that" but that is not what you are saying. You are saying: "I love and respect you enough to accept that this is the way you are right now and that you are doing the best you can. Even if the way you are is not my preference"

You may have ties with teachers from your early school years. Perhaps you've become just like one of them. Examine what might have disturbed you about them.

Young children are so impressionable and reactive - they accept what is told to them as the truth. They have yet to learn to "read between the lines" with people. Eventually they become so fearful of becoming like others, they become preoccupied with it and neglect their own development. There is an extraordinary being inside each of you that is crying out to be discovered! Do you hear your soul calling out to you? You are the only one who can free it from its chains and its isolation. Your soul needs to evolve, to breathe and to have space to grow!

By letting others dominate you with their attitudes, you unconsciously become more and more like them. If you did not accept authority, it dominated you. By developing a grudge toward authority, you became more authoritarian, or controlling in your own behavior. You decided, without even realizing it, that in order to survive, you needed to try and control what was going on around you. You became imprisoned by that decision.

As you continue to hold a grudge, your ego grows. You believe that you've been treated unfairly. You will carry this around with you at an enormous price! This "chip on your shoulder" will be costly in every relationship you become involved in and your health and happiness will be permanently in jeopardy as your body and superconscious mind persistently send you messages that remind you that you are going against the Universal Laws of Love. There is no escape other than FORGIVENESS!

The first step is to FORGIVE yourself for judging the person in question. Then FORGIVE that person for whatever it was you were blaming them for (this is done by putting yourself in the other persons' shoes and imagining why that person did what they did. By doing this, you are automatically forgiving the other. And most importantly, visit the person in question and speak with him. Share your feelings openly (it is not necessary to go into detail). Ask him to FORGIVE you for being blind to his way of loving and explain what you had been blaming him for that caused such an obstacle in you.

If the person is deceased, sit by yourself in a quiet room and relax every part of your body. When you feel totally relaxed, imagine that you are sitting next to that person. Talk to them - tell them how you feel and ask for their forgiveness. Even if you are not in contact physically with that person, their spirit is there. You may find this exercise to be quite emotional, but it is very cleansing. Don't be afraid to open up and get in touch with your feelings.

When carrying a grudge, you imprison both of you by tying you together. This cord drains energy from both people, spiritually, and will cause mental and emotional exhaustion. When you free yourself, you will automatically free the other. You will release them to their own space and energy and will allow both of you to grow and evolve. You will help him grow further, even if he is deceased, by releasing him from the bonds of your ill feelings.

If you approach the other person with the expectation that they will feel sorry for you, you are not cutting the cord. If you hope to hear: "Oh, poor you! I never realized I made you feel that bad!", you are not coming from your heart. You are expecting the other person to take responsibility for your emotions, even though it was you who decided that he did not love you in the first place. Nobody can make you feel angry or sad. It is your decision to feel angry or sad.

Observe what you are feeling when you are talking to the other person. Are you expressing your feelings with the purpose of learning how to love them, or so that you will be understood by them? Simply SHARE your feelings with the other person. Whether he understands or agrees with you is not important. You are doing it to free yourself - it is for your sake alone. When you hesitate to do so out of fear of hurting someone, or of possibly being misunderstood or laughed at, it is a signal that your ego is taking over...and you'll be left right back at step one. You will continue to be locked into your suffering and stagnation. Fear will keep you from being free.

If you are the oldest sibling in the family, you may have more ties with your parents than the others. The first child is always the one with the least space because the parents usually have higher expectations of their first-born. Once the second and third child are born, parents have become more realistic. This leaves the oldest child dealing with greater parental expectations and demands that he may have resented or not met.

In many cases where a parent would have preferred a child of the opposite sex, is because that parent has not enjoyed their life so far and thinks that it would be a burden for the child. Knowing that your parent had that desire, you might feel rejected, but you don't have to. The desire had nothing to do with you, they simply wanted a better life for you than they had.

Be strong. Look at one situation at a time, cut one cord at a time, and eventually you will be free. You don't have to do it all at once, but with practice, each cord will become easier to cut.

One common issue is the attitude toward money. For most of our parents, money was of prime concern - it had to be "saved". Their happiness was often dependent on the material aspect of their lives - money was synonymous with security. Happiness was a direct result of financial security. They wanted you to have money so that you would be happy. That was their way of loving. If you are inclined to be a little extreme with your saving or spending habits, you are probably reacting to your parents' attitude.

The Universal Law of Love dictates that parents and children love each other. It is impossible for it to be otherwise. The love between parents and children is profound and precious - remember that your soul made a conscious decision to be with your parents. You knew then what you would have to learn from them and that the more difficult the lesson, the more valuable it would be. Keep that in mind as you unearth each of the ties and understand deep in your heart how much your parents really loved you, regardless of the situation. You chose each other for a reason.

Once you have managed to cut the ties, you will have learned to love and respect your parents for who they are and who they were. You will have forgiven them and asked their forgiveness ... you will feel an extraordinary sense of well-being and inner peace. A tremendous weight will have been lifted from your shoulders and you will feel light and free as a bird.

If your grudge has grown to hatred, it is critical that you attend to it. The energy produced by hatred is the most destructive and toxic energy there is, whereas love's energy is completely healing. To live with hatred in your heart will alter your body chemistry, triggering violent and painful diseases. Hatred destroys its master. In fact, laboratory studies have proven that the breath of a hateful person, when administered to a rat, was sufficient to kill the animal instantly. Each hateful thought can be compared to swallowing a mouthful of poison - without exception. The cord built on hatred is so strong that the efforts needed to cut it will have to be much greater and more sustained. This is because a hateful person is further removed from his love center than most.

CHAPTER 6 EXERCISES

» On a sheet of paper, write down everything you can remember that bothered you about your parents during your early childhood and adolescence (from birth to approximately 18 years old).

» List the things that bothered you about other people who influenced you during the same period.

» Choose one of the situations listed and go through the process of accepting responsibility for your part in it. Using the same situation, see the love that was underlying. Then, go to them in person and express what you are feeling. Forgive them and ask their forgiveness.

» IMPORTANT - It is essential that these exercises be done before going on to the next chapter. You may find that a lot of emotions will surface. Don't be afraid - you are opening doors that will lead you to your freedom.

» Repeat this affirmation as often as possible:

I FORGIVE EVERYONE I JUDGED AND I NOW BREAK FREE FROM THE TIES THAT PREVENT ME FROM BEING IN HARMONY WITH MYSELF. I LOVE MORE AND MORE WITH MY HEART.

» If there is someone with whom it is especially difficult to feel love, here is an affirmation that will help you open your heart:

I FORGIVE (name of person) COMPLETELY,
REGARDING (situation or attitude in question) AND I
WANT ONLY GOODNESS FOR HIM/ HER
THEREFORE, I FORGIVE MYSELF FOR HAVING
THE SAME ATTITUDE, FOR I BECOME WHAT I
JUDGE.

CHAPTER 7

FAITH AND PRAYER

What is "faith"? Faith and "belief" are often confused. "To believe" is defined as "to accept as true". If you think that what you believe is the truth and it makes you happy (and if it is of benefit to you) then live by it and share it with others. Those who agree may accept it as their truth - those who disagree will not. Truth, however, is in perception and is not absolute, so it will change according to one's own beliefs.

Faith, although more fundamental than belief, is much broader. The Scriptures define faith as "the confirmation of our hopes and the evidence of the unseen". When you are motivated by faith, you trust in a knowledge that is not limited by your own belief system. You know, deep in your heart, that there is a much bigger picture and you are convinced that you will get what you deserve and desire from the unlimited resources provided by the Universe.

Almost two thousand years have passed since JESUS delivered his message of love and faith to the world. It's time we started living according to his profound and vital teachings. To have faith is to have an unshakable trust in GOD's presence within ourselves. We were taught to pray by saying "GOD, help me". In saying this, we are referring to our inner GOD. HE does not exist "somewhere out there, governing the Universe from afar", but within the hearts of every living being. When you see yourself as a living manifestation of GOD and when you feel His great power within you, you can achieve anything you desire - such is the power of Faith.

Here is a story I like very much, as it clearly illustrates the concept of faith:

A small town was experiencing the effects of a serious drought one summer and the farmers were concerned for their crops. One particular Sunday, after mass, they asked the priest for advice. "Father, we must do something or we will lose our crops". The priest replied: "All you have to do is pray with absolute faith. A prayer without faith is not a prayer. It must come from the heart". That week, the farmers gathered twice a day to pray for rain. The following Sunday, they visited the priest. "It didn't work, father - we got together every day and prayed but there is still no rain." The good priest asked them: "Did you really pray with faith?" They assured him they had. The priest added: "I know you did not pray with faith because none of you walked in here this morning with his umbrella!"

When we have faith in our hearts, there is no question whether or not we will obtain our desire. We often practice faith unconsciously - for example, merely switching on the light when we enter a room is an act of faith. We don't question that there will be light.

When you order a new car, you decide on the model, the color, the accessories, and you sign a contract with the dealer. "Don't worry", he assures you, "your car will be here in six weeks, just as you ordered it. I'll give you a call the minute it's in!" This is an act of faith. During those six weeks, you have faith that the car will be delivered exactly as you ordered. You begin to notice the cars on the street that are the same model and you say: "That car is just like mine!" You have no problem visualizing yourself behind the wheel. You wanted the car, you took action by ordering it and you will clearly have it, just as you envisioned. You had faith in that vision and you made it happen.

You can achieve anything you want quickly, asking only once, if you have faith that the result is already there. When you ask for the same thing more than once, it is because you are uncertain that you will receive it. The power of faith will help you turn your dreams into realities. Be patient and KNOW that they will be manifested.

If you formulate a general affirmation without much energy, you are praying. If you formulate it and visualize it clearly at the same time, you have faith. Imagine it with clarity, feel the result and it will be yours.

JESUS said in the Gospel (St. Mark): "Everything you ask for when praying, believe you have already received it and you will see it come through." "Everything is possible for the one who has faith." FAITH CAN MOVE MOUNTAINS.

In understanding your connection to the Universe, to your inner GOD, you will understand faith. Take a look around you. When you see the harmony in nature, still untouched by man, you can't help but marvel at a magnificent sunset, the vastness of a powerful ocean or the peace of a starry sky. The Universe is in harmony -in synch with its own pulsation everywhere you look. The sun rises every morning, the moon shines every night, the planets dance their dance and the tides keep time to the rhythm of the Universe. There is a Divine plan - you can feel it in your soul. There lies faith. Embrace it and live your life as it was intended.

It is all there for the taking; this is our Divine heritage. You need only ask. GOD has given you free will, to live your life as you wish. You have the right to all the riches of the Universe (except, of course, what belongs to others). If another person has something you would like, ask GOD for one of your very own.

The Law of Abundance assures that billions of us benefit from the sun, the air and all of the riches of the earth. The same law applies to material riches. Divine Heritage is Universal - material wealth exists for all of us. YOU HAVE A RIGHT TO RICHES! You need only claim your share of the heritage.

The only difference between you and someone who is well-off materially is your degree of faith. He believed it was possible to achieve what he has achieved. You need only do the same.

Faith does not come from the mind - it comes from your superconscious mind, which is your inner GOD. If you were to visualize your inner GOD as the sun, faith is a ray of sun that links you to Him. Contrary to reason, faith accepts without asking how or why. When we have faith, we have absolute certainty. Although we may be unable to see it, we know without a doubt that what we desire already exists and that we can make it happen in the visible world.

ALL OF MAN'S GREATEST ACCOMPLISHMENTS ARE THE RESULT OF FAITH. The one who wants to "see it" before he "believes it" has no faith. If all human beings felt that way, mankind would have accomplished very little.

Every time you say: "When I have this or that, I will be happy ... I will be able to...", you lack faith. Step one: acknowledge what you want. Step two: take action. Step three: know that you have achieved it. If taking a holiday with your family would make you happy, show that you have faith by making reservations for your trip. Once you have decided that you will make it happen, go and make a deposit at the travel agent. You will be well on your way. All it takes is an act of faith.

Divine Law states that the sun will rise in the morning and that when you sow beans, you will reap beans. To achieve what you desire in life is just as natural. You possess within you the same power that is exhibited in Divine Law. It is natural for the power of GOD within you to manifest whatever you envision.

GOD is like electricity in that it is a great natural power that we cannot see; we do not know where it comes from and we do not understand its workings, nevertheless we know it exists. If it is dark when you enter a room, does that prove that there is no electricity? No it is only that you have not turned on the light. Each act of faith is a switching on of the light - the more faith, the more light; everything becomes clearer.

Do you see how simple it is? All you need to do is touch the switch. You need not understand the source of electricity or how it works...you need only touch the switch. By accepting GOD's energy in you, it is manifested through you. Use it freely and wisely.

Everything that exists in the visible world originated in the invisible world. Whether it is a building, an airplane or the clothes on your back, the initial thought took form in someone's mind. You have access to this creative power. Whatever mankind conceives already exists in the invisible world - he has used his mind to tap it and his thoughts to bring it forward.

Once the thoughts are made clear, all that is needed is action to manifest it in the visible world. It is an elementary process.

By nurturing what you have created in your mind, you will radiate the vibration needed to attract the right people into your life. You will know what action to take and you will find the right place in which to materialize this thought. This also works in a negative way. If you visualize something negative for yourself, it also will materialize itself. Use your faith to produce positive experiences: there are a multitude of them within your reach and more than enough for everyone. It is up to you to claim your share.

If, for example, there were unbelievable stockpiles of wheat just waiting to be claimed. Whether or not it was claimed does not change the fact that it was there for the taking. You only have to dip into the reserve!

Don't waste any more time! Start NOW to utilize your power by developing your faith. Start NOW to create happiness in your life so that you can share it with others. YOU CANNOT GIVE SOMETHING YOU DON'T HAVE. If you are filled with doubt, fear or worry, you cannot possibly be sharing happiness with others - you can only share doubt, fear and worry. Start loving and taking care of yourself and allow beautiful things to happen to you. Automatically, you will be sharing them with others.

When you take a trip, you know your destination and whichever means you choose to get you there, whether car, train or plane, you are confident that you will arrive at your destination. If your destination is inner peace, let yourself be guided there. Have faith that you have everything you need within yourself to get you there. Let go and surrender to your faith. Ask and you shall receive.

Once you have more faith in yourself, you will discover that you have more faith in others. It's a marvelous discovery! You will no longer be influenced by negative people once you realize that everything happens inside of you, rather than outside of you, and those of faith will be drawn to each other. With their combined positive and faithful energy, the dawn of a new era of love will be upon us.

JESUS taught us about faith with the following words:

"Do not be concerned with food, water or clothing. Isn't life more important than food and your body more important than your clothes? Look at the birds; they do not sow or harvest, have no storage room or attic and nevertheless our Heavenly Father nourishes them. Are you not worth as much as they? Why torment yourself about clothing? Look at how the lilies grow in the fields. They do not work or spin; even Solomon in all his glory was never as richly dressed. If GOD looks after a flower that will be cut tomorrow, how will He look after clothing you, man with so little faith! No need to ask yourself "What will we eat, drink or wear?" Only heathen worry about that. Your Heavenly Father knows your needs. Look for GOD's kingdom and His justice and the rest will be given to you in addition. Do not worry about tomorrow, because tomorrow will look after these things by itself. One day at a time."

These words from Jesus invite us to live in the here and now. Nothing good comes from worrying about tomorrow. By accepting that you have the power to fulfill your needs as they appear, you will always achieve your goals.

There is no need to accumulate a fortune for your old age, nor do you need to stockpile insurance. In being preoccupied, as such, with your security, you are exhibiting fear and insecurity. You believe that any power you have now to obtain money will be lost when you reach old age. You accept God's power in you now, but believe that it will not be there in the future. Instead, have faith that when you are older your wisdom and experience will help you obtain and accomplish anything you desire -even more easily than you are able to now. Why accumulate excessively? It is more important to have what you need right now.

Being present in the moment - being grateful for THIS moment is what is important. It is said that "SUCCESS CAN BE MEASURED BY YOUR DEGREE OF APPRECIATION". By being truly thankful for everything you receive each day, you will continue to receive everything you need. Worrying blocks the flow of abundance and lies as an obstacle in your path. Nurture only beautiful thoughts and your life will take a wonderful turn!

CHAPTER 7 EXERCISES

» TAKE A LEAP OF FAITH. Choose something you have wanted for some time and decide RIGHT NOW to make it happen.

» If you need to put a deposit down on something material, on a vacation package, whatever - do it. If starting the ball rolling entails making a phone call to someone, do it.

» DO IT WITHOUT FURTHER DELAY! In life, "being" should always precede "having". If you are thinking "When I win a large amount of money in the lottery, I will buy the house of my dreams and then I will be happy", you are going against natural laws.

» Don't wait until (fill in the blank) to be happy. Be happy first. Then take action. You will have what you desire.

» Repeat the following affirmation and go on to the next chapter.

I BELIEVE IN THE GREAT DIVINE HERITAGE WITHIN ME AND I DRAW FROM IT EVERYTHING I NEED WHENEVER I NEED IT.

CHAPTER 8

ENERGY

Do you have enough energy to make the most of your day or would you like to have more? Most of us would give anything for a little more energy! Researchers in California discovered that the human body has, potentially, enough energy to light a city like Montreal or New York for a whole month!

Nothing creates energy like POSITIVE ANTICIPATION! Motivation and satisfaction generate tremendous personal energy that fuels you to realize your goals. This energy will make all the difference in your quality of life!

Here's an example: A young lady, coming home after a long exhausting day at work, is so drained of energy that she doesn't even feel like preparing a bite to eat for herself. She lies down on the sofa for a much-needed rest. Her physical and mental exhaustion are very real. Just then, the phone rings and a gentleman friend that she is especially fond of is on the other end of the line. He tells her that he will be over in half an hour to see her. What do you envision? That's right - she's never run so fast or been so mentally alert as she hides dirty dishes, makes her bed, rearranges her apartment, hurries to the corner store for just the right bottle of wine, freshens up (and has never looked so good). When he arrives, she is glowing - full of energy and life and will likely dance the night away. MOTIVATION CREATES ENERGY!

Running out of energy is a signal from your body and your superconscious mind that you are not living in harmony with yourself. You are cutting yourself off from the source and expending energy without recreating more. You are depleting your energy resources and only what motivates you will replenish them.

THE ENERGY CENTERS

The physical body is surrounded by an invisible and more subtle body called the etheric or vital body. This body is composed of a magnetic energy field that looks like thousands of small lines surrounding the physical body. At seven precise locations in the body, twenty-one of these lines converge to form areas of energy called "Chakras".

THE BASE CHAKRA is located at the base of the spine. It is the seat of physical strength and survival. You tap into this energy when you experience rage, pain or fear. When you experience insecurity regarding your survival, worrying about food or shelter, you directly affect this energy. These emotions cause an imbalance of energy at the base chakra. Too much energy concentrated in this area could provoke lower back problems. This chakra interacts directly with the adrenal glands which produce the correct balance of cortisone and adrenaline needed for your physical body. Thus, by experiencing insecurity, fear or rage, you are wasting this energy when you could be doing something much more constructive.

THE SACRAL CHAKRA is located behind the sexual organs, between the pubis and the navel. The Sacral Chakra is the area from which all sexual and creative energy is generated. Reproduction, or the creation of new life, is the primary function of the sexual organs. This area also affects the flow of energy to the Throat Chakra, which represents creative expression. When the energy in this area is inadequate or overly concentrated, both the Throat and Sacral Chakras will be affected. This energy is also used for all sexual activities and for the expression of passion, hate, anger, ego, jealousy, selfishness and possession.

When possession, jealousy, anger or hate take over in your life, it is an indication that you want power over others. In doing so, you drain the energy meant for your sexuality and your creativity, which will manifest as problems in the sexual organs or as swelling in the lower abdomen (as much for women as for men). Once you learn how to rid yourself of these destructive emotions, alter your behav-

ENERGY

ior and master your ego, you will find that a great deal of energy will rise up to your throat and will help you develop talents and gifts and create abundantly. You will communicate more freely and with confidence.

THE SOLAR CHAKRA is located between the navel and the heart. It is the area of emotions and desires. When you experience strong emotions or desires, are bothered by them and do not express them, you are blocking this area of energy. Thus, your energy is blocked and there is a lack of energy circulating throughout your body. This explains your lack of energy whenever you experience guilt, frustration, aggression, sadness or other negative emotions. When the energy becomes concentrated and blocked in the Sacral Chakra, it affects the pancreas and the entire digestive system which are directly connected to this area.

Any fear or insecurity is funneled directly into the Base, Sacral and Solar Centers and held there as blocked energy. It is vital to have this energy circulate to the spiritual parts of the body.

The first two centers represent our animal instincts. The Solar Center is situated between the instinctive and the spiritual centers. The first three centers are linked to "having" and "doing", the other four, the spiritual centers, to "being".

THE HEART CHAKRA is located in the heart region. It is the source of love and compassion, which means it is critical that this center be kept open and functioning. It affects the thymus gland, which develops immunity to disease. Unfortunately, many people have blockages in the heart chakra, caused by a surplus of emotional and intellectual energies. When the heart region closes, it jeopardizes the immune system. As you learn to accept full responsibility for your life, to master and to express your emotions fully and to love unconditionally, your energy from the Solar Chakra will rise up and fill the heart. The more energy that can circulate freely from bottom to top and top to bottom, the more you will be able to utilize its power to accomplish whatever you desire. Each act of love creates a

ENERGY CENTERS – CHAKRAS

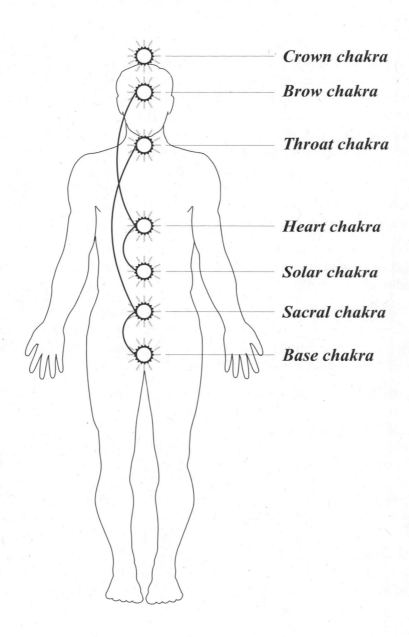

Crown chakra

Brow chakra

Throat chakra

Heart chakra

Solar chakra

Sacral chakra

Base chakra

small opening that allows a better circulation of energy at the heart level.

THE THROAT CHAKRA is located in the region of the throat. It affects the thyroid gland, which in turn, controls the entire nervous system, metabolism, muscular functions and the production of body heat. The Throat Chakra is also the center of all expression, including creativity.

It is connected directly to the Sacral Chakra, which houses the tremendously powerful sexual energy that fuels our creativity. This energy is expressed also through the throat. If your creativity is suppressed or not expressed truthfully, you are not utilizing your creative power to its full potential. Deficiency of this energy in your Throat Chakra will result in sore throats, voice problems and laryngitis and may also affect the thyroid gland.

To maintain harmony in the Throat Chakra, remain true to yourself in thought, word and deed and express your creativity in alignment with this truth, whether through music, art, literature or nature. Your creative force will also be carried over into your work, your hobbies, and most importantly, in the manifestation of your life's desires.

By being persistent in your efforts, you will reap great rewards. Very few people are true to themselves 100% of the time, but it is possible. Get started in that direction! In order to be true to yourself, what you think, say and do must be in alignment. This center is called the "freedom doorway". When you have learned to be true and to love with your heart, your energy will circulate freely and travel to the higher spiritual centers.

THE BROW CHAKRA is located primarily above the nose, between the eyebrows. It aids in the development of the Third Eye. It is the source of psychic gifts, paranormal powers, intuition and clairvoyance. Its main function is to develop your true nature.

Individuality starts in the Throat Chakra. The last three chakras (the throat, heart and solar) represent a person's true nature, or individuality. Following the paths of others will cause you to lose touch with your own individual nature. Only in finding you're own essence will you become your own master.

THE CROWN CHAKRA is located at the top of the head. It is the center of illumination and enlightenment. Its high vibrational frequency is the source of the halo surrounding the heads of saints and very spiritual beings that often appeared in religious paintings. When this center is developed fully, that person experiences the "I AM", or total fusion with GOD. Jesus, Buddha and many other spiritual leaders reached that state of perfection and bliss.

The top two chakras (the brow and crown), can be further developed through the practice of meditation and service to others. This service must be carried out with a pure heart and humility, with NO EXPECTATIONS and through unconditional love. This is the only kind of love for mankind that enables one to become a great spiritual being.

Human energy comes from many sources: the water you drink, the air you breathe, the food you eat, the thoughts you create and the activities of your etheric body (the latter being your main source of energy).

Previous generations in our culture were unaware of the ability to generate energy from their thoughts. This is why their need for food was greater. The more a person's thoughts are pure and true, less food he needs. When the etheric body is harmonious , energy circulates freely and provides a pronounced intake of energy that is only exceeded by one's need for air and water.

Everything is composed of energy - it must always be in balance, even while being utilized. If you continuously give to others while refusing to receive, you will not find inner harmony and balance. There must be a balance in the circulation of energy. Pouring energy into the accomplishment of your desires will accelerate their realization. Those who expect to receive anything without an output of effort, or energy, are ignoring natural laws of physics. A relationship that exists where there is an uneven exchange of energy will not last

very long. Both partners must contribute evenly in order to comple-
ment each other and keep the energy of the relationship balanced. In
this way, neither is dependent on the other and both will grow. The
same holds true in relationships between parents and their children;
there must always be an even exchange of energy. I'm sure you have
found this to be true in your own experience.

Living in a home that was given to you will never give you the
same joy and meaning as a home you have worked for, or even built
yourself. The more energy you put into it, the more you will get out
of it.

It is unfortunate that some people feel "the world owes them a
living" - that everything is due them without any expenditure or effort on their part. It creates tremendous imbalance. Here is an example of what I mean: A young handicapped woman sits in her
wheelchair, nursing a grudge she has against a society that will not
provide her with everything she desires. She wants it all and expects
the government to take care of her. She is isolated in her wheelchair
and feels helpless to do anything about her situation. She is psychologically and physically immobilized. As long as she fails to realize
she is solely responsible for the realization of her goals, nothing will
change. She will feel worse and her handicap will continue to limit
her.

She is too busy spending her energy on negative feelings, blaming society and GOD for her situation. Taking matters into her own
hands would empower her to achieve whatever she would like to
achieve.

CHAPTER 8 EXERCISES

» Take a good look at your everyday life. Do you feel that you are
   depleting your own energy resources for others? Do you give
   them all your energy, having none left for yourself? If you do, it is
   because you are not giving freely, but have expectations. You

probably have difficulty asking for and receiving help from others, which creates stress and a sense of dissatisfaction in you.

» If this is occurring in your relationship with your children, it is because you are giving of yourself without daring to ask for anything in return. You are afraid of hurting them or disturbing their lives in any way. You do not want to "intrude". You must change immediately! Talk openly to your kids - tell them that it's important to have an equal exchange of energy between you and that you must "be there" for each other if you all are to succeed. This will create a synergy that will begin to multiply the rewards for all of you!

» If your energy is being depleted at work or with your mate, it is up to you to bring about change by openly discussing the matter with whoever is involved. Take care of yourself regardless of what others may think or feel about it. You are doing it for yourself, but everyone around you will benefit.

» Once you have understood how to increase and balance your energy in every area of your life, proceed to the next chapter.

» Here is your affirmation. Repeat as often as possible:

I AM MORE CONSCIOUS OF MY GREAT ENERGY AND AM RELEARNING TO USE MORE WISELY.

PART TWO:

LISTEN TO YOUR PHYSICAL BODY

CHAPTER 9

DISEASES AND ACCIDENTS

I don't know what the words "disease" and "accident" mean to you, but most people seem to think they are the result of misfortune or bad luck; that they are manifestations of injustice in their lives, especially if the disease is "hereditary" or contracted through someone else. This way of thinking is contradictory to the Great Universal Law of Responsibility.

The concept of self-responsibility, when it pertains to accidents and disease, may seem a little extreme to you, but we cause them to happen unconsciously. That's why it is difficult to believe that we are thus responsible for them. An illness is simply a message sent to you by your body. It is a signal given to you by your superconscious mind, or your inner GOD, to tell you that something in the way you are thinking or behaving is going against the Great Universal Law of Love - the Law of Responsibility. To blame nature or to be angry when you become ill is senseless. Instead, be open to the message that your body is giving you and thank ROUMA for it. When you do not completely understand what it is telling you, ask it for guidance - for clarification -so that you can understand the message and accept it fully and find the peace of mind you will need to heal yourself. Accept your inner GOD.

"Why is it I still have such a bad cold?" you ask. "I am so tired of being sick! I've had enough - I never feel well any more!" or "I have another migraine!" or "My back is killing me...!" With such affirmations, you are refusing to take responsibility. Ask and your superconscious mind will answer you. Unless you are open to receiving this information from your superconscious mind, you will continue to suffer from diseases and accidents because you will not be alert to their causes. Once you have clearly heard and understood your message, you must act accordingly to bring about your healing.

Here is an analogy: It is dark and your neighbor knocks on your door to inform you that you have left the lights on in your car. You ignore him, but he continues to knock and do whatever he can to attract your attention. He sincerely wants to help you, but you think that he is bothering you. If you ignore him completely, you will eventually find that your car battery has died.

Your superconscious mind acts the same way with you. If you ignore or misunderstand its signals, it will continue to send you more. This will go on until, eventually, you will develop cancer or have a serious heart attack - whatever it takes to shake you up and alert you to make changes in your life. If you still choose to ignore the message at that point, you will end up like your car battery.

Doesn't it make sense to become a little more attentive and sensitive to what your body is telling you?

If you simply thanked your neighbor for warning you about your car lights, put on your coat and immediately went to shut them off, you would be solving the problem. If you tell your neighbor you will take care of it, but don't bother, he will be back again: "I guess you didn't understand me the first time." Your superconscious mind does the same with you. Through its repeated messages, it prods you into taking action.

Isn't it extraordinary that you have this friend inside of you that loves you unconditionally - one who guides you consistently toward health and happiness - one who is there exclusively for you? Embrace him and be grateful for him -he will never let you down.

Whenever you experience physical discomfort, your body is giving you a signal. Illness is never just physical - it is the physical manifestation of a metaphysical (beyond the physical) message. The seriousness of a disease is a direct correlation to the seriousness of its message. If it is a powerful disease, it has been building in strength for a long time. Your soul is screaming for help - it is time to become reacquainted with the great healer, LOVE.

Here are some common illnesses and their metaphysical causes:

ARTHRITIS

If you suffer from arthritis, it means that you are convinced that someone is taking advantage of you, but you keep your suspicions to yourself. Arthritis affects people who cannot say "no" and blame others for taking advantage of them. In actuality, others react according to the vibrations they receive from you; they take advantage of you because you unconsciously invite them to. The message your body is sending you through arthritis is: "Stop thinking that everyone is taking advantage of you...you are the one saying "yes" when you want to say "no". Assert yourself. Say no when you really mean it. When you choose to be of service to someone, do it, but do it without expectations and with joy in your heart. Stop trying to change others - become more in tune with your true nature."

KNEE PROBLEMS

Problems with the knees indicate that you are stubborn and inflexible. Very often, it is a sign your ego is strong and dominates your thinking. It is the sign of an authoritarian person who wants to control others because they are insecure. they hold stubbornly onto their ideas. If you have a sore knee, the message is that you should be more flexible and stop concerning yourself with what others will think of you. Accept the opinions of others. Is there someone in your life that you are frustrated with because they don't agree with you? Let go and let them be who they are. Your body is telling you to stop contradicting the Law of Love.

MOUTH

Problems in the mouth indicate fixed opinions. Your mind is closed and you refuse to acknowledge a message in the opinions of others.

TEETH

If your teeth are causing you problems, it indicates indecision. You resist making a decision for fear of the outcome. You are currently required to make a decision regarding something important in your life and your body is telling you: "Don't be afraid - whatever you decide will be fine, it comes from your inner knowing."

GUMS

If your gums hurt, it means that you have to reinforce your decisions. You are being told: "Don't be afraid - now that you have made up your mind, act accordingly."

BACKACHE

Any problems in the area of the back are an indication that you feel you are carrying "the weight of the world on your back". You feel that you have no support and that you are responsible for the happiness or misery of all your loved ones. Your superconscious mind is sending you the following message: "Stop thinking you are responsible for everyone else. If you want to give others support, don't do it out of a sense of obligation, but of your own free will." Take responsibility for your own decisions - you will be able to handle them.

When a person feels he is lacking support from others, he wants it, but usually will not allow them to give it to him out of pride. Eventually others become discouraged and no longer offer further assistance.

If your pain is in the UPPER BACK, it is related to lack of support from others. LOWER BACK pain is an indication of lack of material or monetary support.

FEVER

Suppressed anger results in fever. The only outlet the body can find to express it is through a bout of fever. Too many locked-up feelings and desires are exploding. Your body is letting you know that you must communicate your needs, rather than keeping everything to yourself. Choking back your anger is not beneficial to you. You are only punishing yourself.

ARMS

When there are problems in the area of the arms, it is a result of underestimating your value or your usefulness. You feel unappreciated and worthless compared to others. Your body is sending you the following message: "Be conscious of your purpose wherever you are - you are needed and appreciated." Problems with the arms may also indicate that you are presently afraid to seize an opportunity that is of benefit to you. It may also indicate that you are dissatisfied with what you do for a living (metaphorically - "what you do with your hands"). Do you need a career change? Make a note of when your arms are bothering you. You are being told: "Go ahead - don't be afraid to do what you find fulfilling."

LEGS

You need your legs to move you forward - thus, problems in the leg area indicate a fear of going ahead - fear of the future. Your superconscious mind is there to let you know that you need not worry. You are inherently capable of accomplishing whatever you desire. If, for example, you are deliberating over a career change but are concerned for financial reasons, the pain in your leg is telling you that now is the time to go ahead with your plans without worry.

THROAT

Many people claim their sore throat is due to a cold or an abuse of their voice. The throat is the instrument of expression. Your superconscious mind is telling you to express yourself, which you are presently afraid to do. You are withholding your expression or hiding your anger about something. You were probably disturbed by some remark or may have been so surprised or insulted that you were unable to answer back right away. You swallowed your words instead. You were unable at the time to hear the love or suffering behind the words that were flung at you. Often, we are not even conscious that some words have hurt us. We would rather believe that words have no affect on us because it is less threatening, but we are very vulnerable to words. Your soul knows you have been hurt, thus your throat is hurting. The action necessary to alleviate this pain is to approach the person in question and, without accusation, express what you experienced when these words were said.

LARYNGITIS

If you suffer from laryngitis, not only are you afraid of expressing yourself verbally, but you are especially afraid of voicing your opinion to someone in authority. To avoid his reaction, you prefer to "swallow" your opinion. Don't be intimidated by others. The person you are speaking to will appreciate both your concern and your honesty. If your laryngitis is hiding anger or a grudge, you must free yourself by expressing it openly. I suggest you say "Right now, I am afraid of your reaction. I do not want to hurt you, but I must talk to you. I need to do this for myself - I need to express my opinion." If you delay, you will only store your negative feelings deep inside you. Persistent or reoccurring laryngitis indicates that you are not listening to the message your body is giving you to express yourself.

BEDWETTING

The child fears one of his parents very much. It could be either parent or someone else who is taking over in a parental role. The fear is not necessarily of anything physical - it may be that the child loves the parent so much that he fears displeasing him. The child will constantly be on his guard and will never be free to be himself. It is important for both parent and child to understand the psychological implications of bedwetting in order to get past it. Ensure that the child understands that he is loved unconditionally and need not fear retribution of any kind. He will relax and no longer have to live with the anxiety of displeasing his parent. You will notice a big change in his outward appearance, too - he will become more confident and radiant, knowing he is loved just for himself.

COUGHING

Someone who coughs constantly is someone who feels suffocated. He experiences an ongoing anxiety and nervousness and feels "jammed" by life. On the other hand, a temporary or occasional cough is a sign of criticism or boredom. The cough occurs at the very moment the person is feeling annoyed or criticizes himself or others inwardly. His body is trying to tell him: "Please stop criticizing or being annoyed. Instead, try to relax and accept the present situation."

INTESTINES

The way the mind assimilates and digests ideas is mirrored in how the body assimilates and digests nutrients. Constipation occurs when you hold on to old ideas and refuse to make room for new ones. It is often the sign of a closed mind, pettiness and greed. You do not make room for new ideas and you probably hold on too tightly to material possessions. Your superconscious mind is telling you that it is time to let go of the past.

Diarrhea means the opposite. Letting new ideas slip away too quickly, you reject them, indicating a fear of the future. You wish situations in your life could be resolved quickly so that you wouldn't have to deal with them. Diarrhea often indicates rejection of oneself, or fear of being rejected by others. The body is sending you the message that you don't have to be afraid. Fear is a manifestation of the imagination. The body only receives a physical signal when your fear is not beneficial to you. Fear that is experienced, for example, when crossing the road and suddenly realizing you are in the path of an oncoming truck, is healthy fear. There was a real danger to your well being. The other kinds of fear are not.

KIDNEYS

Kidney problems affect people who are critical and who are often feeling disappointment and frustration. They constantly feel victimized and trod upon. Such thoughts are very negative and create unhealthy body chemistry. Your superconscious mind is sending you this message: "You are responsible for everything that happens in your life - accept that responsibility now!"

BREASTS

Breast problems are indicative of an overly authoritarian attitude toward someone, which is not beneficial to either one concerned.

EARS, EYES AND NOSE

Eye problems indicate that something you see is bothering you. It is probably none of your business. That is why your body is talking to you. If, on the other hand, it does pertain to you, take the necessary steps to change the situation. The same phenomenon is indicated when the problem is in the ears. You are being disturbed by something that you have heard. When the nose is involved, the body is telling you that you are upset by the way you "feel" about someone or something. In regard to the eyes, ears and nose, the body is telling you that you needn't be bothered by others - LIVE AND LET LIVE.

ACCIDENTS

Having an accident is an indication that you are feeling guilty about something. Human beings have an automatic reflex to punish themselves in order to neutralize guilt. For example, when peeling potatoes, you may start thinking to yourself: "Oh, I've forgotten something again - what an idiot!"...and you cut your finger. You may think that you cut yourself because you were preoccupied and were not paying attention to what you were doing, but, subconsciously, you were punishing yourself for being "such an idiot".

As soon as you feel guilty about something, your body lets you know - whether through a small incident or a big accident. An accident is a warning and its message is: "It's time you became aware that guilt is unconstructive and useless. Wake up." This may seem a little extreme to you, but take a moment to look back at some of the incidents and accidents you have been involved in and you will see how closely linked they are to your own feelings of guilt.

Taking a closer look at the metaphysical reasons for physical discomfort and disease, you will become aligned with the principles of the healing process and gain control of your own health.

In my second book (soon available in English), which discusses the metaphysical meanings of many specific diseases, you will find a complete description of the metaphysical correlation of many physical diseases. Ways to help you discover your own personal causes of disease will be discussed further.

When doing the exercise for this chapter, you will begin to understand that every physical discomfort, disease or accident that you have experienced is nothing more than a warning or a signal from your superconscious mind. It will stop the minute you acknowledge your body's message and act on it with love and positive anticipation. It takes no more energy to stop it than it did to create it! Your energy was merely incorrectly channeled. Once your illness has subsided, you will notice an increase in your energy level.

A persistent illness indicates that you want to have power over someone else; possibly your illness is allowing you to receive attention that you crave and would not receive otherwise. If that is the case, find out who it is that you want this attention from and resolve it some other way, for the sake of your own health!

There is one thing in common with every message your body is sending you, and that is "Stop wasting your energy on negative thoughts - everything always works out for the best."

CHAPTER 9 EXERCISES

» Draw up a list of all your current physical discomforts.

» Thank ROUMA for sending you signals regarding these discomforts and ask your superconscious mind what their meaning is.

» Take care of at least one of these discomforts. Take the smallest one, if you wish, and make it disappear! Having done so, you will understand the correlation between the physical and the meta-physical.

» Repeat this affirmation as often as possible and go on to the next chapter.

I TRUST MY BODY, WHO IS MY GUIDE AND MY GREATEST FRIEND, MORE AND MORE EACH DAY. IN DOING SO, I REGAIN PEACE, HEALTH, LOVE AND HARMONY.

CHAPTER 10

FOOD FOR THOUGHT

The physical body is the most extraordinary machine ever imagined! No human being has ever been able to develop anything remotely similar in function and efficiency. In theory, if we were to build a computer that could assume all the functions of the human brain, that computer would be the size of the earth itself. Presently, human beings only utilize between 5% and 10% of their brain capacity.

The human body knows instinctively, from the point of conception, what its requirements are. It does not have to be taught how to sleep, be thirsty or hungry, cry, cough, perspire, be warm or cold, eliminate, digest, yawn, vomit, swallow, laugh, move, bleed or heal itself. Somehow, in the process of maturation, we've forgotten to trust our instincts.

A mother trusts the instincts of her newborn baby. When he expresses hunger, she feeds him, she soothes him when he is upset and knows the meaning of his cries...yet, as soon as the first teeth appear, she decides he is ready for three meals a day. After only a few months of life, we've stopped trusting the innate intelligence of this child.

He learns from this early age to nourish his body according to someone else's decisions. By listening to someone else (his mother), he will be prevented from remaining in tune with his true needs. By the time he is fully grown, he will have lost touch with them almost completely.

There is an interesting correlation between our eating and drinking patterns and the way we lead our everyday lives.

How do you feed yourself? Do you have a fixed routine for your meals? Do you eat unconsciously, without asking your body what it needs at the time? We are so programmed to eat a certain way, that it doesn't occur to us that there may be another, even better way to do it.

It reminds me of a young bride who cut both ends of the ham off before placing it in the baking pan. Puzzled, her husband asked her why she did that. She answered: "I don't know - my mother always cooked ham that way." Curious, the young man asked his mother-in-law why she also cuts both ends of the ham. She answered: "I don't know - my mother always cooked ham that way." During a family gathering, he asked the grandmother the same question. She told him: "You know, young man, when I was young, my family was very poor. We only had one pot and it was much too small for the whole ham, so we had to cut both ends." This story illustrates how much thought we give to the way we are doing things. We are creatures of habit, living virtually unconsciously.

How important are habits and traditions to you? Take a look at your eating habits. If you are like most North Americans, you probably eat at regular hours every day out of routine. You have been taught that "three meals a day" are standard procedure. You are also afraid you will become too hungry if you do not eat regularly. If you are going out for the evening and fear your dinner may be later than usual, you may have a bite before you leave. You are worried that you might be hungry later. So out of fear, you eat now even though you are not hungry.

Your body knows very well when it is hungry. It can function without food for weeks without any ill effects. If you feel hungry two or three hours before having a chance to eat, talk to you body this way - "Please wait, ROUMA. It will not be long. I will feed you soon." Never concern yourself with under or overeating, if you are listening to the signals your body gives you. You may think you're hungry and getting a signal from your body but the signal is from your mind, it is only out of habit.

If you discover that you are someone who has many eating habits, you may also notice that you are the kind of person who is very concerned about what others think, do or say about you. Instead of thinking, acting or dressing in a way that pleases you, especially if it is considered "unusual", you tend to be more concerned about the reaction of others and will conform so that you do not initiate any kind of negative response. Worrying about such insignificant things can be draining on your energy and will create an underlying dissatisfaction inside you. Learn how to be conscious of your real needs.

Eating by habit will also show you that you are probably very rigid in your judgment of right and wrong and are dogmatic about your opinions. You decide that this is wrong and this is right when, in fact, there is no right or wrong. What may seem wrong to you may seem right for someone else. Let go of what others are thinking and doing in their lives, regardless of whether you think they are making "good" or "bad" decisions. I cannot stress enough the importance of "LIVE AND LET LIVE" - let others live their lives the way they need to and get on with your own. Get in touch with what YOU need inside to make your life a success!

Eating patterns often emerge strictly out of habit,which stem from the mental dimension, but it is more common to develop emotional eating patterns.

As a young child, food was used as a form of love or compensation. Even today, you probably find yourself offering cookies or candy to a child who is upset, just to soothe him. Children are manipulated with food. For example, a parent will say: "If you're a good boy, I'll take you to a restaurant"...or "we'll go for an ice cream". An even better example of manipulation with food is: "If you're not a good boy, you'll have no dessert!"...or "no snacks until you finish your homework". What a barrage of mixed messages your body is receiving! It came into this world believing food was meant to nourish it - now it is being taught that food is a tool used by adults to manipulate our behavior! What an impact this must have on our emotional selves. How you reacted to this manipulation as a young child will shed some light on how you function as an adult. Whatever left the greatest impression on you between the ages of birth and seven years regarding food, has left its mark on your mental, physical and emotional dimensions (The imprinting of your early eating behaviors and habits). Your reactions to this imprinting will give you the clues to get to the root of your current reactions to food.

What can you determine from your current eating patterns? Do you drink or eat out of boredom, to kill time, to soothe or reward yourself - or do you often find that you are eating for emotional gratification? (In a later chapter, I will deal with mastering your emotional eating patterns.)

Satisfying the senses is another reason for eating. This is eating with "appetite" (Webster defines "appetite" as the natural desire for satisfying some want or need especially for food). Appetite does not stem from hunger. For example, the smell of popcorn, whether you are hungry or not, is almost irresistible to most people. When your senses consistently have the upper hand, you can get yourself in some trouble. In another example, you may be walking along the street and come across an ice cream parlor. Suddenly, you have an irresistible craving for ice cream and you begin to salivate when you see the variety of flavors. Again, the senses are ruling your decision. But, if you are sitting at your desk one morning and, all of a sudden, you are craving a pastry, that is not appetite. It is a desire. It was not set off by any of your senses. You wanted that pastry before seeing it, smelling it or even hearing about it. Make sure that you are really hungry and if the answer is no, then the desire for the pastry was maybe set off for an emotional reason.

There are many other things you can do by appetite. You can shop by appetite, sleep by appetite, make love by appetite, etc. Observe yourself a little. What do you do by appetite? Do you have difficulty mastering your senses? If the answer is yes, your physical dimension is not mastered. It is not in harmony.

Once you notice that you act by appetite, it is that you are receiving a message from your God Self. Rouma is telling you that one or many of your senses are psychologically unsatisfied. It can be sight, hearing, smell, taste or touch.

SIGHT

You are letting yourself be bothered by something you are presently seeing. Your body is telling you: "What is bothering you is none of your concern - none of your business"... or "do something about it instead of being annoyed - resolve it."

HEARING

Something you hear, whether at home or elsewhere, is bothering you. Do not judge, but resolve it.

SMELL

Is there someone or something that you just can't take anymore? It could be a friend, a family member, a co-worker or even a piece of furniture.

TOUCH

You're not getting enough affection? Who forgot to sow some? You only reap what you sow. Affection can be expressed in many simple ways - a kind word, a card, flowers, a love note or a smile. It is also very important to show yourself some affection. Remember, start sowing some and you will reap some.

TASTE

If you are eating out of appetite, it may be that your sexual appetite is not satisfied. It is up to you to bring about the necessary changes.

Whenever one of your senses is dissatisfied and it concerns you, take action. If it involves someone else doing or saying things contrary to what you would like, your body is telling you to mind your own business, let the other person do what they have to do and concern yourself only with your own needs. It is very dangerous to let one's happiness depend on others.

Whichever dimension has the most hold over you, you must master it. If it is the mental dimension, start questioning why you do things the way you do - you are living on auto-pilot. Before doing anything, ask yourself: "Does this make me happy? Is it in my best interest? Is this really what I want to do, say or think?" Wait a few moments and the answer will come to you. You will begin to feel more satisfied with your life if you become more aware of what you are doing and why.

If your life is ruled by the emotional dimension, learn how to express yourself openly. (More about this in Chapter 18).

If your physical dimension rules, stop and ask yourself: "Which one of my senses is not satisfied?" Go through them one at a time and identify which one is not being fulfilled. Take a good look inside yourself - your body knows.

Using this method of identifying the reasons for your behavior, you will discover some interesting things about your inner self. You will realize that you may function on all three levels (physical, mental and emotional), but that one dominates. Once you get in touch with this concept, you will find that your eating patterns will change - you will tend to eat because you are hungry, rather than for emotional reasons or out of habit. Your taste in food and clothing may actually change as you transform your thinking and become more in tune with your true nature.

Your body never loses sight of its fundamental needs or its true nature. Learn to listen to it. Chemically, it is composed of six essential nutrients: water, proteins, vitamins, glucides (sugar and carbohydrates), lipids (essential fats) and minerals. Each time one of these elements is out of balance, your body gives you a signal by sending a message to your brain. Your brain passes that message on to you by making you hungry or thirsty for something specific. Once you learn to communicate with it clearly, you will be able to provide the correct nutritional balance required to keep you in optimum condition.

You see, you need never worry about whether you are getting enough food or the right kind of food, if you learn to listen to your body. Trust it to tell you exactly what you need and when you need it. Never eat when you are not hungry "in case you don't get a chance to eat on time..." Wait for the signal from your body - it will tell you what is required in terms of nutrition when a deficiency is indicated (i.e.: iron, calcium, protein, fat, sugar, etc.). It will ensure that you have a taste for precisely the food that will balance you. Your brain, the ultimate computer, has registered the chemical make-up of every food you have ever tasted and knows exactly what to prescribe.

The physical body has a responsibility to notify the brain of its needs. It is not the role of the mind. For example, someone who is on a "diet" is dictating to his body what and when it is to eat. This goes against nature. When on a diet, you send the following message to your body: "As of today, I will decide what you need, when you need it and how many times a day I will give it to you." Do you think you know your own physical needs better than your own body? LEARN TO TRUST YOUR BODY!

Some people only require one meal a day - some, only breakfast. Many prefer breakfast and supper -no lunch. Other people need to "graze", or eat many small meals throughout the day. It is up to you to discover what suits you best. Each person is unique. What is beneficial for one may not be for another.

It is imperative that you are aware of how your body functions. Some people assimilate calcium with difficulty; some have difficulty eliminating cholesterol. Being unconscious of the needs of your particular physical body will cause some difficulties. Eventually, you will reach the point in your awareness where you will know what is going on in your own body. The superconscious mind, through the physical body, controls digestion, assimilation and elimination, but it is your responsibility to help your body in any way you can.

As you increase your level of awareness, it will be easier to recognize and interpret your body's messages and act accordingly. Do your share and your body will do its share. In this way, your energy will become balanced and more evenly distributed. Being in harmony ensures good health.

Many people continue to use certain ingredients in their daily diet that do not provide nutrition for the body and only cause the loss of energy. Among these poisons are alcohol, white sugar (and other refined foods such as white flour, white rice and white bread), caffeine, salt, tobacco and all chemicals (medicine, drugs, preservatives and colorings) as well as non-essential fats. There are many good books on nutrition available on the market. I would suggest you consult your local library or bookstore, if you are interested in investigating the subject of nutrition further.

Be aware of what you are feeding your body. If you have not already done so, start now to provide a balanced nutritional program for your body and you will find it will be a matter of a few weeks before its chemistry stabilizes. Respect it and take care of it. In doing so, balance and harmony in the mental and emotional dimensions will follow suit.

Body chemistry is determined on a cellular level and is affected by the balanced or imbalanced interaction of all three levels - the physical, the mental and the emotional. Eating foods that are difficult for your body to digest or that include poisons, shows disrespect for the body. For example, a meal of smoked meat with fries, salt and dill pickle is hard to digest and contains toxic components that disrupt and poison the body. If you force your body to ingest alcohol, soft drinks, sweets and chemicals, it is a signal that you do not like yourself very much. Don't be surprised when your body can not do what you ask of it and you are robbed of energy. Your body is your best friend -you are in this together. Treat it accordingly.

Craving sugar is an indication that you lack sweetness in your life -you do not allow yourself things that would please you and when you do, you feel guilty.

Cravings for salty foods indicate a critical, judgmental personality. You are probably your own worst critic.

Cravings for spicy food: your life is probably more bland than you would like.

Caffeine cravings indicate a need for stimulation on a psychological level.

Look inside yourself for a moment and ask what it is that you need to do to satisfy your need for stimulation or excitement, rather than continually pouring more of these things into your system.

CHAPTER 10 EXERCISES

*Note: I would strongly suggest that you wait one week before going on to the next chapter. Re-read Chapter 10, paying attention to everything that you eat and drink during that week.

» Every day, ask yourself if you are really hungry before eating or drinking anything and ask your body if it is what it needs. At the end of each day, write down what you were feeling and what was going on at each meal, or snack - did you eat out of hunger, habit or for emotional reasons? This exercise is not for the purpose of creating a "diet plan", but to help you become more aware of what dominates your life - what part of your life needs to be more balanced - the physical, the mental or the emotional. Once you have determined this, you will find you are more in tune with the needs of your body and better able to provide them.

» Here is the affirmation:

I AM MORE AND MORE ALERT AND CONSCIOUS OF WHAT MOTIVATES MY WAY OF EATING AND I NOW WAIT FOR MY BODY TO LET ME KNOW WHAT IT NEEDS AND WHEN IT IS HUNGRY.

CHAPTER 11

THE IDEAL WEIGHT

In discussing weight problems, both overweight and underweight are equally important issues. To be abnormally thin indicates that there is not enough emphasis on your material life. Your lack of weight reveals the presence of a certain amount of guilt whenever you admire material things, or when you would like to please yourself materially.

It may also mean that you spend too much time worrying about the world's problems. You are easily worried - you question everything that happens around you and are depleting your own resources by taking on responsibility for the behavior of others.

Thirdly, it may be that you give more than you receive. You must learn to accept the bounties of life for yourself. As you transform your attitude about your own worthiness, your weight will become more balanced. It is important to let your body function with its own rhythm. Listen to it.

The opposite problem- being too heavy, or gaining weight too easily - indicates several things. When someone "goes on a diet", he shows a fundamental lack of responsibility in his life. He wants to alter the effect without determining the cause . Success from dieting is only an illusion; that is why it is usually only temporary (statistics indicate a 98% failure rate of permanent success) . The body reacts when it is mistreated. Most people gain back more than they have lost.

Remember that your body, through your superconscious mind, is your best friend. It communicates with you in many ways. Instead of thanking it, you rebel; you want to change it because it does not coincide with the image you want to project. By communicating with your body , you will get to the root of the problem and weight loss will become a simple, healthy process. The rate of weight loss will vary with each individual, but by identifying the cause, you will ensure that you will reach your ideal weight when it is most comfortable for your body. If it took you many years to gain twenty pounds, you can't expect to lose it in a couple of weeks. Give your body the time required to adjust to your transformations inside. As you change your way of thinking, the rest will follow.

Because gaining excess weight is due to several causes i.e.: eating out of habit or from emotional or sensual deprivation, your approach to weight loss must address your specific motivation.

Eating more than your body requires, nutritionally, will result in an accumulation of fat. This manifestation, however, is not automatic for everyone. It is one of the ways that your body is able to send you a message. I'm sure you know someone who eats excessively without ever gaining a pound; they have a higher metabolism than most. This means that the calories they ingest are burned at a faster rate and that the digestive system is continuously activated. As a result, that person will likely burn out more quickly and age more rapidly. We all have our own inner messages. The body, our best friend, always finds a way to communicate its needs to us.

To circumvent any problem, it is best to eat when hungry and to stop eating when comfortably full. This practice alone would induce weight loss! Listen to your body - you will receive all the signals you need. Act on them.

Excess weight is often the outward expression of accumulated ideas and thoughts, not only material goods. One who accumulates too much of anything is afraid of being without. It is this underlying insecurity that causes people to be overweight. It also is the reason people accumulate a lot of insurance - for fear of being without. They are usually very attached to their material goods. This kind of attachment is detrimental to your spiritual growth and evolution. Learn to let go and trust that you will always have enough.

Perhaps you would like to own a lot of material things, but won't admit it even to yourself. You secretly dream of having more. Here is the message from your superconscious mind: "It is your birthright to be surrounded by beauty - material things can be very spiritual."

Excess weight may indicate a lack of acceptance or lack of love of oneself. You feel you are unlovable, unworthy, and crave the acceptance and love of others. You are afraid of being rejected, but rejection is only an illusion. You will receive as much love as you give. Look around you - you will realize that you are loved more than you thought.

Sexual frustration or refusal to accept one's chosen gender are also causes of obesity. If one or both of your parents would have preferred a baby of the opposite sex, you may have believed, from birth, that you were unwanted. This could have a tremendous influence on your life-long sense of acceptance. If you were of the opposite sex, do you really believe life would be easier for you? Have either one of your parents ever complained about the problems and obligations of being male or female? Those sexual frustrations often have lasting repercussions that begin in adolescence. Teenagers can be very intimidated by someone of the opposite sex. They can also feel very insecure with the authority of a person of the opposite sex. They begin during adolescence to neglect their physical appearance to avoid having to attract and deal with the opposite sex. This commonly results in obesity.

If this is so in your case, your superconscious mind is telling you to accept your sex. Whether you chose to be male or female, it was because you needed to learn the lessons that only your chosen gender would experience in this life. Accept your sex and you will be much happier; by not accepting it, you become removed from your true self.

Obesity may also be a manifestation of a "tie" that needs to be cut with someone. When you were younger, was there someone in your life who was overweight whom you were unable to accept? By entertaining the fear of being like that person, you have succeeded in creating the very thing you feared. There is a lesson to be learned here about acceptance. Look inside yourself and come to accept and love that person as he was, physically, mentally and emotionally. You will then find you can accept yourself and your weight problem will no longer be an issue.

It may be that there was someone in your life when you were younger whom you loved and admired - and he or she happened to be overweight. If you admire the qualities of that person, accept them for yourself without taking on the physical characteristics.

Weight problems that have been with you since birth may be caused from something in a past life. Just like someone who was born handicapped, this particular handicap may be necessary in order to learn the lessons needed in this lifetime. Learn to love and accept yourself THE WAY YOU ARE. You will have to go through life this way until you understand the message you are being given or the cause behind the physical, mental or emotional handicap you are dealing with. It has happened that a handicapped person miraculously experiences a complete recovery - usually accompanied by a profound spiritual revelation. The same phenomenon applies to weight problems. No one has to go through his whole life putting up with "karma" from a previous life. You alone can decide when to put a stop to it.

Many devout and spiritual people have weight problems because their souls vaguely remember dimensions other than the earthly one and long to be elsewhere. Those people often seem to have their "head in the clouds." Unconsciously they aspire to being in a better place. They may not be consciously thinking about suicide, but a part of them would prefer not to be here. By carrying excess weight, they are more solidly anchored to earth. The message is as follows: "Please accept, once and for all, your presence on earth. You have a purpose here - you have to learn to love and accept yourself and others." If this is your case, concentrate your attention more on nature and see the beauty around you. Begin to love yourself and accept your place in the universe.

In the case of excess weight, it may be that you are receiving more than you are giving. Are you afraid to reveal yourself to others? Perhaps you have built a wall around yourself because you feel too vulnerable. Do you share your thoughts and feelings openly, or do you feel that others should experience the same pain and "learn the hard way" like you did? Take a close look at why you keep everything inside you -are you afraid of hurting someone else or of not being accepted and loved for who you are? Are you the kind of person who enjoys other people's secrets and problems, but wouldn't dare share your own? Find the courage to shed your emotional baggage and you will also shed the physical baggage.

Your superconscious mind has a million ways to talk to you - so become aware of what it is saying and how it is telling you. These messages may show up as acne, redness or rashes on the body, visible or invisible diseases. Learn to detect them.

Look at what is going on inside you - get to the cause and the effect will take care of itself. Diets are not the answer - they are only a Band-Aid and they are contradictory to the natural flow of the body. When someone has a problem with alcohol, he drinks to forget his problems. The next morning, the problems are still there, and they seem magnified by a terrific hangover.

Dieting leads to the same result. Even if you are successful in losing weight temporarily, the underlying cause is still there and will bring you continuing inner dissatisfaction. Go directly to the cause and deal with it, if you want to succeed in achieving and maintaining your ideal weight.

Remember: don't be concerned with the length of time it may take to achieve your weight loss goals. Learn to follow your body rhythm. What is most important is that you are learning to become master of yourself and, ultimately, your own destiny. So...forget words like "diet" and "cheating" when dealing with your weight loss. Nobody cheats in his life. If you believe you are cheating, it is because, inwardly, you are still on a diet and you are letting your mind govern your body's decisions.

Instead, when you feel you've "cheated on your diet", ask your body for forgiveness. Say: "Excuse me, ROUMA, but I have been abusing you. I have given you too much food - I didn't listen to you. I'm doing my best; be patient with me -we'll get there together." Working alongside your body, like a good friend, will keep you from feeling the unnecessary guilt that often accompanies a "diet".

CHAPTER 11 EXERCISES

» Make a list of all the foods you deprive yourself of presently. On this list, include the foods you would like to eat or drink but don't dare to for fear of putting on weight. Acknowledge that there is a part of you that is still "on a diet".

» Accept the idea that you can eat what you want and when you want. IT IS YOUR BODY. You do not owe an explanation to any-one but yourself.

» Begin to listen carefully to what your body is telling you that it needs. Try to be aware of any "cravings" you experience and de-termine their basis. Before you eat anything, ask yourself if you are really hungry and if that particular food is beneficial to your body. Eat consciously.

» Remember that programming yourself with "cannot" and "should not", will only cause obsession and will push you to achieving the opposite of what you want to achieve.

» Repeat this affirmation as often as you can and go on to the next chapter.

I ACCEPT MYSELF AS I AM RIGHT NOW. MY GREAT INNER STRENGTH IS HELPING ME REACH AND MAINTAIN MY IDEAL WEIGHT.

CHAPTER 12

SEXUALITY

Sexuality has always been a delicate topic. Surprisingly, even in this day and age, few people truly accept their sexuality. Because of the number of deeply-rooted psychological and spiritual factors that come into play through sexual expression, it is a difficult and complicated subject. Our sexuality is primal and fundamental to our very being. Through our sexuality, we have the potential to express our innermost selves and this element alone causes most people a great deal of discomfort.

From generation to generation we have retained the fears and guilt associated with the word "sex". It wasn't that long ago that "sex" was still synonymous with the word "sin" - especially in the Catholic church. Confessionals were opened so that sins could be openly admitted and redemption sought, but thoughts about sex or sexual acts were simply not mentioned. We carried the guilt of having committed these "sins" and the guilt of not admitting them! That's pretty bizarre, considering that sex is the fundamental, biological act of procreation - the very act that ensures continuation of the species!

The sexual act is the physical expression of the greatest possible fusion - that being the fusion of the Soul and the Spirit. A human being's fundamental purpose lies in achieving the fusion of his lower body with his higher body. This is why the sexual act is such a large issue. The Soul has a profound need to reach fusion with the Spirit - an act that culminates in profound bliss.

For this reason, we have high expectations of the sexual act on a deep level, but are disappointed and frustrated on a more material level. This frustration and misunderstanding about sex is what is transferred from one generation to the next. Parents hinder the sexual development of their children by passing on the hang-ups and patterns of sexual behavior they have experienced. Because sexuality is not properly understood, there is a dichotomy that results in obsession and denial...the ultimate recipe for guilt!

A relationship based solely on sex is deprived of a solid base. The longer a couple develops a friendship prior to engaging in sexual intercourse, the more solid the relationship will be.

Sexual problems, both for men and women, are numerous and the results are indicated by the vast number of sexual diseases. Menstrual problems are an indication that the female is in some sort of denial of her sexuality. Menstruation is a natural biological function of the female body and need not bring discomfort. We were created perfect. would never have created anything to suffer.

Human beings harbor tremendous sexual energy that cannot continually be channeled into sexual performance. It is the ultimate creative force and it is essential that it be recognized and used as such. Earlier generations did not understand the power of sexual energy and were much less creative. Their lives were monotonous and uninspired in comparison to more recent generations. That is why they were so preoccupied with sex. They, however, were frustrated in its expression and the energy became bottled up.

Life today offers more avenues of expression of this fantastic energy. Take a look at our youth - they are certainly expressing themselves in their clothing, their hairstyles and their overall demeanor. The difference between then and now is the acceptance of that expression.

Girls usually have more guilty feelings related to sex than boys do. It is still not acceptable for females to bare their chests publicly, but it is more acceptable for males. Females are not quite safe alone at night, lest they might be sexually assaulted. Girls get pregnant, boys don't; the consequences of sexual expression are more severe for females than for males.

Numerous sexual taboos exist at the unconscious level. We must get rid of them, for by stifling our full expression, we will be prevented from attaining fulfillment and inner peace. As a child, we made important decisions about sex that carry over into adulthood. If a child catches his parents having sex, his attitude about the sexual act could be very much influenced by their reaction. If they punish him "for looking", or if they try and hide themselves, they are giving him the message that there is something wrong with what they are doing.

The Oedipus theory comes into play when a child is between three and six years of age. At that stage, children are becoming aware of their sexual energy; the little boy falls in love with his mother and the little girl with her father on all levels, including the physical. The little boy may become jealous of his father - a part of him admires his father but, on the other hand, he wants to take his father's place beside his mother. He feels caught between these two conflicting sets of feelings. Allowing a little boy to continue to sleep with his mother at this stage can be confusing for him. It is time to gently explain that he is "a bigger boy now, that he has his own room and that the parents have theirs."

A little girl at this stage may also exhibit very sensual behaviors toward her father. She kisses and caresses him frequently and will interfere if he pays too much attention to her mother. This stage is normal and healthy, but must be dealt with carefully, without discouraging normal development. I strongly encourage parents to talk to their children openly about what is happening to them, without giving too much detail. Children understand more than we give them credit for.

The Oedipus complex gradually disappears as the child nears six years of age. By this stage, both boys and girls have developed a new respect for the parent of the same sex and jealousy is replaced by admiration. The child identifies with the same-sex parent and develops a mentor bond that replaces any jealousy that formerly took place.

Many sexual problems in adulthood stem from an Oedipus complex that was never properly resolved. Women will continue into adulthood seeking their father and men go on to search for their mothers. If this behavior is far too familiar to you, don't be too concerned. All you need to do is recognize it and cut the tie. Accept your parent as your parent and not your lover. Paternal or maternal love and intimate love are two vastly different things. Confusing the two has been the cause of rampant incest. I must admit that I am astonished to discover that one in five people who come to my personal growth school reveals a history of incest! An enormous number of people are dealing with this trauma. Thankfully, it is acceptable to discuss this openly in this day and age, so that these psychological wounds can be healed.

What is the reason behind incest? A young girl is not conscious of the sensuality she radiates and the fact that she is provoking a reaction in her father. The father is then left entirely to bare the blame for not controlling himself and ultimately traumatizing the child. However, he does not completely understand what is happening to him. What he is doing goes against a natural law. Because of his immaturity on a sexual level, he is susceptible to the vibration that exists between him and his daughter. This type of man is often afraid of being rejected by women and was not given the opportunity during his upbringing to mature sexually. His sex life with his wife is unsatisfactory and it is easier for him to get satisfaction at home rather than going somewhere else. His chances of being rejected are less. Often his family life is very important to him.

My work enables me to work with and get close to a great number of people -many of whom have had incestuous experiences. Most of them blamed the father. Remember the Great Law of Responsibility. We always reap what we sow. On a subconscious level, we are responsible for what happens to us.

I know of many cases in which the incest began at a very early age and continued up to 18 years of age. Under these conditions, do you really believe the father is the only one to blame? A young woman revealed to me that she was terrified of her father and the only way she could get what she wanted in terms of her social life, etc. was to do "what her father wanted". Do you think that, at 18 years of age, she was unable to say "no" in that situation? Something more is going on at the unconscious level.

The problem generally stems from the child's basic need for love which, by remaining unmet, becomes disproportionate. The young girl adores her father, but does not feel he returns her love. When he expresses it sexually, she is initially grateful for the contact. She begins to feel guilty once she realizes this type of contact is inappropriate. She also may carry some guilt about taking her mother's place.

It is typical of the spouse of an incestuous man to prefer to ignore the situation, most often unconsciously, out of fear of having to face the truth. Therefore, the young girl often hates her mother for not being able to see the truth and for not doing something to protect her. On a subconscious level, the child knows the situation is causing damage. It is common for the spouse of an incestuous man to have had some incestuous experiences herself when she was young and is confused and afraid herself. She can't face what is happening.

Incest between a mother and son occurs much less frequently, but the experience is much more traumatic for the child because the "mother/child" tie is destroyed. A mother symbolizes the source of all life. By losing that source, the child feels totally lost.

If you have lived through such an experience with your father or with someone else you trusted, it is very important for you to forgive that person, to forgive yourself and to accept that it was not unnatural for you to enjoy the sole form of love you received from them. The hatred and sense of violation that is often subsequently propagated is like poison in your life and benefits no one. In this situation, forgiveness has a powerful impact (see chapter 6).

It is vital to cut this tie in order to put a stop to the vicious circle of guilt and condemnation that undermines your self-worth. The purification must start somewhere - you can bring about such a transformation. UNDERSTAND THAT THERE ARE NO VIOLENT OR WICKED PEOPLE - ONLY SUFFERING PEOPLE.

The sexual act should only be experienced out of love. In loving someone, you desire union with that person for the purpose of fusion. Sexual intercourse should never be used as a bargaining tool. Thousands of women SUBMIT to their partners, believing they will get something in return.

When entering into a new relationship, it is important to start on the right foot. Do not use sex as a way to create a bond because this will usually undermine any healthy bonding. If your relationship has already been established on a stable footing, over a reasonable period of time, talk openly with each other about your sexual interests...how you feel about it and what you felt about it when you were younger.

It is important to learn to be open about sex. Have you ever taken the time to sit down with your partner and go into the details of your first sexual encounter? Do you remember the person, the date, the place...? If not, it may indicate a sexual block.

Making love when both partners are in love is the most rewarding and fulfilling experiences on earth. Sexual desire is the Soul expressing its need to merge with the Spirit.

Having sex is the symbol of the spiritual fusion with our God Self. It allows your superior body to bring you great inner joy during sex and afterward. One experiences a profound inner peace after making love with someone they are in love with. This is certainly no place for judgment or guilt! Making love is not animalistic unless you do it only for the physical pleasure it brings you. At that moment, only your lower body is functioning.

It is important to make love with a partner that you have chosen carefully. A woman receives a great deal from the man during the sexual act, just as the man receives a lot from the woman. Not only is there a sharing on the physical level, but on the emotional as well (through the "astral body"). That is why it is essential to know the partner well. If that person harbors ill feelings against someone, such as hatred or fear, you may become affected in the transferring of your partner's energy to yourself. Both the man and the woman receive vibrations from each other through the connection of their energy bodies, the invisible bodies, so be very selective in choosing a partner.

Homosexuality has its origin in an unresolved Oedipus complex. Having fallen in love with the parent of the opposite sex, the normal stage of development, the homosexual goes on to identify himself with the parent of the same sex rather than with the parent of the opposite sex.

There can be many different reasons why a person chooses another person of the same sex as their love and/or as their lover. I sincerely believe that finding "the reason" is not the most important thing. Indeed the most important thing is to use this experience as an opportunity to learn to accept, rather than condemn, oneself.

If you are finding it hard to live this experience, that is, if you feel judged by your family and the outside world, it is an indication that you do not accept yourself. This problem is usually related to the wound of rejection. Rejecting yourself in your sexual preference makes you feel rejected by others and often afraid of being rejected.

Only after reaching total acceptance will you be able to know whether this choice truly corresponds to what your soul needs or if this choice was made in reaction to one or both of your parents. That is what explains why some people live as homosexuals during a certain period of their life and then realize it does not really suit them. Others are and will be homosexuals their whole life. You know you truly accept yourself once you allow yourself to be what you want to be without any fear of being judged by others.

If you are the type of person who frequently judges others for their sexual lifestyle, it is because their choice awakens in you something you have not yet accepted. I suggest you examine what you are judging others for, what you judge them as BEING, and you will discover what it is you do not accept about yourself.

CHAPTER 12 EXERCISES

» Examine your sexuality now and as far back as you can remember. Get in touch with your conscience and try to understand what a tremendous impact your sexuality has on every aspect of your life. Once you understand the connection between your sexuality and your spirituality, your life will be transformed.

» The next time you have intercourse, examine your feelings afterward. Did you accept it for what it was? Was it done out of love? Are your values preventing you from fully enjoying your relationship?

» Repeat the following affirmation often and go on to the next chapter.

I AM A MANIFESTATION OF GOD ON EARTH, THEREFORE MY SEXUALITY IS ALSO A MANIFESTATION OF GOD. I USE MY SEXUALITY TO ELEVATE MY SPIRIT.

CHAPTER 13

PHYSICAL ESSENTIALS

In concluding part 2: LISTEN TO YOUR PHYSICAL BODY, I want you to understand that it is imperative for your own survival that you learn to listen to the signals your body is sending you. Not to do so contradicts natural physical laws. If you become out of synch with your body through non-communication, it will react by manifesting disease.

There are six essential needs of the physical body. They are: breathing, ingestion, digestion, elimination, exploration and exercise.

BREATHING is the body's most important physical need. If you stop breathing, even for a matter of seconds, the result is disastrous! There is no doubt that the physical body cannot do without air. Clean, fresh air contains all the nutrients needed by your body. By breathing properly, the body actually assimilates nutrients from the air by taking the life force, or "PRANA", directly into the cells. Proper breathing enhances digestion, thereby helping the body absorb nutrients from food more efficiently and reducing the need for greater quantities of food. By learning to breath properly, you can actually cut down your food intake by one meal a day!

When breathing properly, take in a deep breath, retain it and take twice as long to exhale as you did to inhale. (If you count to two while inhaling, count to four when exhaling). In this way, you release toxins from the body and clean the respiratory system, which accumulates toxins and waste in its tissues. Eventually, you will increase the count of your breath with regular and sustained exercise. Breathe deeply into the abdomen as you watch it rise and fall. Be careful not to expand only the chest cavity, as your breath will be shallow and, therefore, not cleansing. Concentrate on "filling the belly" with air. As you do so, say this affirmation:" I ALLOW THE

VITALITY OF LIFE TO PENETRATE ME." Each deep breath will bring you closer to a peaceful state of mind.

Just inhaling is not enough to fulfill your physical needs. You must also breathe life itself. Only in being aware of the life force you are breathing will you be able to obtain maximum benefit from your breath. If you are feeling smothered by some of the problems in your life, or if you have lung or breathing problems, you are not inhaling enough of the life force as you breathe. If you reject what is going on in your life even further, you may create heart problems, just as those who take life too seriously and believe that life consists only of hard work and tiresome effort. When you get signals from your heart and lungs, you are not breathing in as much life force as you need. This life force is a primal and fundamental requirement of your very existence.

INGESTION means the taking in of food and water into the body. A lack of food or water result in certain death. I need not convince you otherwise. The quality of water you put into your body is important. Unfortunately, in many cities, tap water is becoming poorer nutritionally. It is said that North America is second only to Mexico for poor water quality. Drink the best water you can, in order to provide your body with optimum nutrition. There are many good bottled waters on the market to choose from.

The quantity of water you ingest is as important as its quality. It is recommended that you drink two to three liters a day to maintain your optimal cellular health. Water conducts electricity and thus determines the quality and efficiency of our own electromagnetic field.

The topic of food was covered in previous chapters.

Have you ever stopped to consider that the meat you eat comes from animals that are herbivorous? How is it these animals became so strong and healthy without eating the meat of other creatures? When eating meat, consider that the animal was frightened when it was slaughtered - he was terrified by the smell of blood in the slaughterhouse and this fear produced a rush of adrenaline in his own tissues. This adrenaline stays in the body and becomes poison for the human who eats it. You are also eating this animal's emotions, as they were stored in his cells at the time of his death. You are ingesting his fear, anger and aggressiveness into your own body. You will notice that vegetarians are consistently calmer than their carnivorous counterparts.

Before putting anything into your mouth, take a moment to listen carefully to what your body is telling you it needs. I am not ordering you to become a vegetarian, if that is not what you want, or to stop drinking tap water completely. My intention is not to frighten you, but to make you aware. Once you become more in tune with your body, your taste for meat will diminish. You will also lose your taste for polluted water. Listen carefully to your body. It knows what it needs and it is your best friend - treat it with love and respect. Remember that your body is also where your soul resides... When you are listening to what your body is telling you, don't shy away from questioning yourself, if the answer seems vague. When you have a craving for something particular, ask yourself if it is really something your body requires or if the craving is coming from some external influence. If after some thought, you still have the craving, indulge it without guilt.

The thoughts we swallow also have a very definite affect on our bodies - as much affect as the food and water we ingest. If you have a hard time accepting new ideas that may be of benefit to you, whether coming from yourself or from others, you may have difficulty swallowing.

Here is an example of one situation that happened to me some time ago: I was in a meeting where important decisions were being made. One of the decisions was related to the future of my personal growth school. Someone in attendance had come up with a proposal that made no sense to me, but I was not too concerned, as the final decision would be mine. Inherently, I had already rejected the idea. As I did so, I began to feel a small ulcer form inside my mouth. My reaction was: "That' strange, all of a sudden I feel a pain in my mouth." A few minutes later, the ulcer had increased in size and I knew I was receiving a signal from my superconscious mind that I was rejecting an idea that would be beneficial to me. By being alert to this signal, I was able to receive profound and unbiased counseling from my dearest friend. I examined the idea that was being presented more closely and with an open mind - I realized that it had many possibilities. Within a half an hour, the ulcer had completely disappeared.

Efficient **DIGESTION** is critical in maintaining good health, whether your body is fed food or new ideas. By accepting a new idea, you have "swallowed" it. If, after doing so, you decide to oppose the idea, saying: "No, it really makes no sense", you run the risk of bringing about indigestion - the rejection of that idea. Your body is telling you that the rejection of this idea is not beneficial to you. Rejecting ideas can cause digestive problems that involve the stomach, liver and pancreas.

The liver is the seat of suppressed anger. To be angry contradicts the Law of Love. *Understand that people are as perfect as they know how to be at any given moment.* Each and every one of their words and deeds expresses their way of loving. By accepting that love, you will no longer need to feel anger and your digestive problems will be over. Digesting new ideas will no longer be a problem.

Problems in the pancreas are manifested as diabetes and hypoglycemia. These two diseases are common among those who do not believe they deserve to be happy. They enjoy pleasing others, but not themselves. Their lives are usually rather dull. They neither accept nor digest the pleasant situations around them and continue to long for a happiness that they need only reach out and grab, if only they felt worthy of it.

Over the years, I have watched many people in my workshops rid themselves of their hypoglycemia through the simple act of pleasing themselves. It may take a little longer to eliminate diabetes, as the disease is more severe and the message is stronger, but nothing is impossible. I myself have witnessed many healings of diabetes.

Chew your food well, until it loses its flavor and becomes almost liquefied. This process aids digestion by giving the stomach less work to do... and the effort to swallow will be minimized. Your body will appreciate it. Saliva contains the enzymes necessary to break down your food. Every time you swallow without chewing properly, even food that doesn't require much chewing, like pasta, soup etc., you make it more difficult for your stomach to break it down. Your saliva contains enzymes for a reason. By taking it a little easier on your stomach and your entire digestive system, you will live longer and your quality of life will be much improved.

ELIMINATION is aided by good chewing and proper digestion. Fiber also plays a key role in efficient digestion, as it acts as a broom in cleaning out the intestinal tract.

It is also very important to know how to eliminate thoughts - to let them go. The pace of our everyday lives causes problems in people who have trouble letting go of outdated and unnecessary ideas.

Elimination is carried out, not only through the intestinal tract, but also through the kidneys and bladder and through the skin. (The skin is the largest organ of elimination in the body.)

Constipation indicates a refusal to let go of old ideas or a fear of losing material possessions. It also indicates stingy thinking. You are hanging onto your thoughts and material possessions too much and are refusing to make room for new ideas. If you have hemorrhoids, your body is telling you that you are afraid of letting go and it causes you a lot of internal pressure. There is resentment and a sense of "overload" in your life. All this discomfort is simply a message from your superconscious mind, ROUMA saying: "You need not fear losing anything - what belongs to you now, you will always be able to acquire." In life, it is a natural law that the more you give, the more you receive - thus the balance of energy and harmony is a given.

Diarrhea is the manifestation of the fear of rejection. Your superconscious mind is suggesting that you let yourself go - open up and let others express their own ideas and let them help you without opposition.

Kidney and bladder problems such as swelling and edema indicate there is a blockage of thoughts and ideas that manifests as blockage in the tissues.

Many skin problems are a sign that the person is blocking his own personality. He controls himself, fearing the opinions or judgment of others. The message is: "Be yourself, let go, don't be afraid of what others might do or say. You have a right to be yourself."

EXPLORATION is a basic human need. This may come as a surprise to you, but one who does not utilize his senses becomes immobilized and his body stagnates until it becomes toxic and death is imminent. If you have ever laid in bed with an illness of any kind, for any length of time, you understand what I am talking about. Human beings need to be active to keep the body functioning!

EXERCISE is vital in keeping the body functioning on every level. Walking is the ideal physical exercise. It is the simplest, the cheapest and the least damaging to the framework of the body. It tends to balance the energy of the body by relaxing and creating a rhythm of movement that soothes and harmonizes. It isolates all the muscle groups, including the stomach muscles, the back, the legs and the upper body. It is wonderful for maintaining cardiovascular health and for cellular oxygenation. Walking speeds up the metabolism, thereby burning calories. It is easy and anyone, any age can enjoy it in almost any weather. It tones body and mind and will reverse the aging process, minimizing the risk of coronaries and arteriosclerosis and by strengthening the immune system. Its automatic movements bring about a sense of freedom in mind and body.

Regardless of your choice of physical activity, for maximum benefit, it should be done an average of four times per week.

MENTAL EXPLORATION is also vital to the health of your physical body. If your actions, thoughts, words and feelings immobilize you and keep you from going forward in your life, you will experience problems in the legs, arms, eyes, ears or nose. Any discomfort in the hip area indicates that you are afraid to go ahead with important decisions. You are aware of what steps you must take, but fear is an obstacle in your path. Your superconscious mind is telling you that it is supporting you regardless of your decision. If the discomfort is in the area of the legs, it is an indication that you fear a change that would be instrumental in reshaping your future. Perhaps a new opportunity has been presented to you and you hesitate to move forward.

Problems in the area of the feet are similar to those of the legs - the toes are related to smaller worries about the future that are not beneficial to you. Worry is never beneficial - "WORRY IS LIKE A ROCKING CHAIR - IT GIVES YOU SOMETHING TO DO, BUT DOESN'T GET YOU ANYWHERE!" A corn on the toe indicates that you believe you have material difficulties.

EVERY ILLNESS IS A SIGNAL THAT YOU ARE THINKING SOMETHING THAT DOES NOT BENEFIT YOUR TRUE SELF.

Pain in the arms indicates you do not embrace your present day experiences with joy. What would you prefer to be doing? It is time to meet your own needs. A pain in the elbow is a signal that you are not flexible in accepting new ideas and experiences. Stop fearing being cornered - everything has a solution.

Arthritis reveals inharmonious exploration. If it is in the hands, legs, arms or hip, you deeply believe that people are taking advantage of you. In actuality, you are failing to express your needs and desires to them; therefore you feel victimized. You sacrifice yourself for others and then complain inwardly about it; your body is telling you that it is time you started asserting yourself.

Your body is extraordinary, is it not? Regardless of what you feel, do, think or say, if it is not for your own, unique benefit, you will receive a signal. Your only responsibility is to remain alert to these signals and to act on them! In doing so, you will be guided to perfection...to LOVE.

I am sure you are aware of some of the indications of the physical needs. In fact, you are probably saying right now: "That's not news to me!" So what are you doing about it? Why do you continue to have many of the symptoms mentioned? Having the knowledge is of little use, if you do not act on it. Many people who accumulate degrees and develop numerous theories regarding these subjects continue to live unhealthy, unfulfilled lives. The reason? They are not putting their theories into practice. They are trying to use their knowledge to impress or change others rather than utilizing it in their own lives.

Having read this far, you are slowly becoming aware of your great inner power and may already be experiencing subtle (or not so subtle) transformation. Go on to the exercises in this chapter.

CHAPTER 13 EXERCISES

» Make a lists of the six basic physical needs. Next to each one, make a note of the signals you have been able to recognize in your own body. It is your responsibility to decide to give your body what it needs. By taking responsibility for your own life, you will learn to please yourself and by listening to your body, you will transform your life!

» At this point, you have learned that it is imperative you remain alert to the needs of your physical body through your superconscious mind. REMAIN ALERT!

» Repeat this affirmation as often as you can think of it.

I AM NOW DETERMINED TO RESPECT THE NEEDS OF MY PHYSICAL BODY AND TO REGAIN MY PHYSICAL HEALTH.

PART THREE:

LISTEN TO YOUR MENTAL BODY

CHAPTER 14

OUR VALUE SYSTEMS

Since the beginning of time mankind has been guided by its notion of right and wrong. Unfortunately, that notion varies from one individual to another and is determined by individual perception. What is determined to be "wrong" is usually based in fear. One person's interpretation of "wrong" behavior, based on fear, can be interpreted as "right" by someone who is not afraid of it.

The truth is, what is often perceived as "wrong" is merely part of the great Divine Plan and exists as a lesson pertaining to the evolution of mankind. Here is an example of variance in perception:

One man, enjoying his early-morning jog in the warm rays of a winter sun, runs bare-chested through the park. For him, for the moment, it is the "right" thing to do. He feels invigorated, vitalized, at one with nature. He is absorbing energy, in spite of the nip in the air, that will carry him through the day. He passes a pedestrian who notices his state of undress and reacts with surprise. The pedestrian comments under his breath "My lord, what a fool! He's going to catch his death of cold!" The pedestrian, had he been running without a shirt, would probably have caught a cold. For him, running in the cold, shirtless, is wrong.

There are unlimited examples of judgments of "right and wrong". It is "right" to eat, in order to fuel our bodies. If it's right to eat, then will we be healthier if we eat even more? Not necessarily. So what determines whether something is right or wrong?

Do you live your life organizing every hour of it based on your concept of right and wrong? How often do you prevent yourself from doing something that you would like to be doing because it wouldn't be right or because you are concerned about what others would say about it? By refusing to do what we know inwardly we need to do, we become out of tune with ourselves. We become creatures of habit, accepting the external influence of right and wrong and structuring our lives around it.

We are told that it is important to "have a good breakfast". "They" say it is best for us. Who are "they"? It may have been pertinent advice when our ancestors were waking at 4:00 a.m. and doing physical work on their farms all day. By 8:00 a.m. they felt the need for a substantial breakfast. Although it may not be common knowledge, even in this day and age, it may be noted that, several generations ago in our culture, people were not aware that they could generate energy through their thoughts. They received energy primarily through their food intake.

Although our lives have changed substantially and our mental processes are more developed than in previous generations, we continue to accept the notions that applied then. For most of us, ingesting a large breakfast only forces the body to digest and try to assimilate what it may not need.

If you find that you are bothered by events and behaviors around you and that you react with guilt, fear, sadness, etc., it is because your mind is telling you it is "wrong". You are out of synch and out of alignment with your true self.

The concept we are fed that Satan is evil and God is good, is an invention of mankind. Once you understand fully that God and perfection are everywhere, you will realize that Satan and its corresponding concept of "sin" are inventions meant to instill fear. Acknowledging evil is acknowledging fear, which is contrary to the Natural Universal Laws. GOD IS LOVE and where there is love, there is no fear.

It is the Law of Divine Order that mankind live in peace and harmony. MANKIND ONLY EXPERIENCES DISCOMFORT WHEN HE LIVES CONTRARY TO NATURAL LAW. Under the Law of Cause and Effect, there is no right or wrong - THERE ARE NO ERRORS - THERE ARE ONLY EXPERIENCES!

The concept of "error" is another human invention, based on what has been fed to us, from generation to generation, in reference to the concepts of "right" and "wrong". What if the words "Satan, sin, wrong, error, cheating " and so on..., were never invented? What if they didn't exist - would you think about them? These examples are a tiny sampling of the negative vocabulary that was developed by human beings and that has been accepted as fact for far too long. Individuals who felt they had knowledge superior to that of Divine Law created their own laws, their own vocabulary, which became one of the pillars they built to support their own POWER.

With the current hunger for spiritual development and inner peace that permeates our planet, we are realizing that it is time to go back to the simplicity of our own natures. The values, methods, habits and principles that have driven mankind to the brink and ruled the lives of every individual, NO LONGER APPLY.

Take a long, deep look at your own set of principles and values. Do they align with your goals? Do you believe them in your heart and do they bring you peace and happiness? The fact that you still feel a need to function according to outside rules and beliefs is an indication that the notion of right and wrong is still too strong in your life. This behavior limits your growth and brings about continuous inner conflict. "I must not..should not..., it's just not right..." is behavior typical of those who cannot let themselves go. They are unable to free themselves of constraint and enjoy their inner child.

Those with strong personalities are usually ego-driven and they all have something in common: they feel a sense of superiority over others, continually trying to change them according to their notion of what is right or wrong. They are under the delusion that they know what is right or wrong and, consequently, have difficulty accepting others just the way they are.

TRUTH IS RELATIVE to the perception of the individual. What is truth to one is not necessarily truth to another. Everyone has evolved to some degree, and everyone carries their own concept of "truth" around with them. No one's "truth" is better or worse or more right or wrong than another's, but it is consistent with the individual's spiritual development. The more evolved a person is, spiritually, the more he will understand that there is no "absolute truth", no right and wrong - only attunement with his own soul. Instead of wanting to change those around him, he will accept them as they are, in their own truth. Each new experience becomes a learning experience, a modification, an opportunity for growth.

When your notion of right and wrong becomes too strong, you become rigid in your judgment of yourself and of others. You lose the "MOMENT", the NOW, by living in a "should have...could have", critical, judgmental frame of mind. All that is meaningful and beautiful in life passes you by as you stand back in judgment. You lose touch with the power and joy of the moment and with the potential vitality that the next moment holds. You stop living. Inwardly, you feel a sense of tension and discontent.

Do you find you become disappointed and frustrated around others who disagree with your opinion on things? Are you not trying to change that person's views? When you do not accept yourself or others, you become angry, hold a grudge and become judgmental and critical. You undermine any possible positive energy. This behavior runs contrary to the Great Universal Law of Love and Acceptance.

You have chosen the way you live and have developed habits based on your beliefs of right and wrong - or have you? Was the decision really yours or were you reacting to the power of an outside influence? What have you based these decisions on?

Sleep patterns are a primary example of outside programming. Take a look at your sleep patterns. Most people maintain consistent patterns - they go to bed at approximately the same time every night, regardless of whether or not they are tired. They get up at the same time everyday, regardless of whether or not they feel rested. Previous generations, primarily farmers, knew a year in advance what their sleep requirements would be. Their lives were set like clocks, yet they knew what their bodies needed to get them through a vigorous work day. Do you want to continue living that way? Do you let the clock tell you when to go to bed?

Times have changed, but sleeping patterns have not. LISTEN TO YOUR BODY! Before going to bed, ask yourself if you really feel sleepy. If so, you may not necessarily need "sleep" - you may only need "rest". Then, choose an activity you consider relaxing...possibly listening to music, taking a warm bath by candlelight, practicing a relaxation technique, going for a walk, solving a puzzle...or even dancing. You know what relaxes you best.

When you are tired, unwind. When you can no longer keep your eyes open, you need some sleep. If you wake up at 6:00 am automatically and roll over, telling yourself that "it's too early to get up", you're not listening to your body. LISTEN TO YOUR BODY. Become aware of your individual needs - don't listen to "them" anymore or to what "they" say. Your body knows what you need. Once you start to listen to it, you will be more invigorated through the day and more rested through the night. Learn to follow your own body rhythms as much as you can and you will avoid the stiffness, backache and headache that often accompany over-sleeping.

Become aware of your habits and begin to question whether or not they are really in your best interest. Here are some common ones: always sitting at the same place at the table, always sleeping on the same side of the bed, going to the same vacation spot, doing the housework on the same day of the week, buying groceries at the same store on the same day of the week, eating and sleeping at specific times, visiting your mother-in-law every Sunday or phoning your mother once a day...even the habit you may have of complaining whenever someone asks you: "How are you?"

Are you used to telling your kids what to do, how and when to do it? Do you have a routine of complaining to your spouse whenever he/she comes in the door at the end of the day? Take a look at yourself. What habits have you cultivated and why?

The more habits you have, the more the notion of right and wrong is ingrained in you. By learning to become more flexible and accepting the idea that there is no right or wrong, you will fill your life with interesting and different experiences that will enrich you and through which you will learn and grow.

Murder, violence, homosexuality, any number of things may be "wrong" in your eyes. Do not judge anyone. Everyone has something to learn from their experiences. It is not up to you or anyone else to decide if these experiences are right or wrong. Only the soul of the individuals involved really know what is going on inside of them and the lessons they need to learn. Those who go against the natural laws of Love and Responsibility will reap what they have sown.

NOTE: YOU REAP ACCORDING TO YOUR INTENT, NOT ACCORDING TO THE ACTION ITSELF. If you reap what pleases you, you know it is because of what you have sown. Learn to stop being hard on yourself by accepting that you are as perfect as you know how to be at any given moment.

Striving for perfection can be a positive thing, but accept yourself as you go. Most perfectionists cannot accept their imperfections. They are never satisfied and have tremendous difficulty with the way things are around them...especially themselves. Nothing will ever be good enough in their eyes. What an unhappy state of mind! Take a look back at what you call your "mistakes". At the time you made these so-called mistakes, were you aware of doing so or did you realize afterward that, if you would have done things differently, you would have achieved different results? My guess is, you were fairly certain your course of action was the correct one - you did your best. So why are you so hard on yourself? Accept that, at any given moment, we are all doing our best. That is what is meant by seeing God everywhere and in everyone.

In some cases, individuals can lose a foothold on themselves and commit heinous crimes such as murder or rape. At the height of their actions, they are not in control of themselves - they are under the influence of some unknown force. Facing and fighting these forces is part of the earthly training for all of us.

The more you learn about mastering your own life, the fewer the events, the less people or outside vibrations will have influence over you. You may have experienced situations where, afterward you had said: "I don't know what came over me -I just wasn't myself."A situation similar to that happens to most of us at some point - it is not unusual. Eventually, however, your own mastery will give you the upper hand in such situations and you will be able to eliminate them. DO NOT JUDGE YOURSELF OR OTHERS - EVERY ONE OF US IS DOING OUR BEST AT ANY GIVEN TIME.

Whenever you hold a grudge against yourself for whatever reason, you are forgetting that you are doing your best. Remember, for example, that a child in first grade cannot possibly exhibit the same handwriting as a university student. The first grade child writes to the best of his ability, It would be like comparing apples and oranges, if you were to compare the two. If, however, someone finds that his handwriting is at exactly the same level at university as it was in grade one, something would have to be done. Always remember that you are "A WORK IN PROGRESS" and be gentle with yourself.

This situation can be compared to someone who has become aware that a specific action contradicts Natural Law but insists on repeating it. Obviously, the consequences for that action will carry a higher price than they would for someone who was not aware.

When doing something to the best of your knowledge, accept that you are as perfect as you can be. The consequences will only become more severe when you knowingly persist in repeating behavior that is not beneficial to you. You must learn from past results. Rarely do we repeat behaviors, consciously, that are not beneficial, but without conscious awareness of our behaviors, we tend to repeat them unconsciously, out of habit.

Every day, every hour, you are presented with opportunities for learning! With each lesson you have a new chance to manifest perfection. Accept this in yourself and you will accept it in others and you will stop condemning, criticizing, judging or holding grudges and you will feel free, possibly for the first time in your life! It's all there for you - take hold of every opportunity and transform your life for the better.

Pessimists and perfectionists usually expect the worst. They accept neither their own perfection nor anyone else's. These behaviors stem from their mind based on their notions of right and wrong. Earth is one big school, progression is continuous from one level to the next; once one level is reached, you do not go backward - only forward. Accept that each of us is at a different level and doing his best according to the level he is at. Some are at the kindergarten level; some have entered university. On Earth, no one is superior or inferior than anyone else.

You see, the university student is not automatically "superior" to the grade one student just because he has progressed further along in his education. They are simply at different levels - there is no reason to judge or to compare. You would be comparing apples to oranges.

When you say: "I have to", you are clearly indicating that the notion of right or wrong has a great deal of importance to you. For example: Perhaps you have put in a full week's work and you get up Saturday morning saying to yourself: "I have to get my housework done today". It becomes a chore - a job to do. You are telling yourself you have no option. Try this: ask yourself if you feel like doing the housework. If not, what would the consequences be? If you decide that you will have no free time to do it during the coming week and that it is important to you that it gets done, tell yourself: "I know I will feel better if the housework is done today." YOU HAVE JUST MADE A CHOICE. You are not doing the housework because you HAVE TO, you are doing it because you have chosen to do so. There is a subtle, but very significant difference in your attitude. You will notice that doing your housework this way will require a lot less energy.

I'm sure you've often said: "I have to go to work today". BE AWARE THAT YOU ARE CHOOSING TO DO SO! You may choose not to go to work, but the consequences may be too severe.

You have made a conscious decision not to pay those consequences and have chosen to go to work instead. This may sound strange to you at first, but think carefully about what I am saying. The difference in your attitude if you make this subtle change will transform the way you approach everything in your life.

Every time you catch yourself saying or thinking: "I have to", stop and tell yourself: "No, I don't have to - I choose to. I don't owe anyone but myself an explanation."

It is your choice whether or not to stop at a red light. If you decide to continue to travel through a red light, you will pay the consequences...perhaps a ticket or an accident; but you ultimately make the decision as to whether or not you will go through the light.

You see, you don't "have to" do ANYTHING! It is always your choice! You must live with the consequences of your decision, but you do make the decision. All that is expected of you in your lifetime is to EVOLVE - to become conscious of your own perfection and to understand that, if you take care of your "self", the rest will follow. By doing so, you will love and act in accordance with the Great Natural and Spiritual Laws.

CHAPTER 14 EXERCISES

» Make a list of everything you consider right or wrong in life. Is your notion of right and wrong consistent with others? Do you assign the same values to yourself as you do to others? Do you do unto others as you would have them do unto you? (Example: do you tell a cashier that she has given you too much change...?)

» Go over the list and determine whether the things on your list are definitely right or wrong, or are they "sometimes right, sometimes wrong", depending on the circumstances, the people involved, etc. In doing so, understand that there is no absolute right or wrong -nothing that applies to everyone, in every situation.

» Make a second list of your habits.

» Over the next three days, change at least one habit consciously. In order to change one non-beneficial habit (such as smoking), you must replace it with a beneficial one of your own choosing. Understand that many of your non-beneficial habits were developed through outside influences - your surroundings, your education, even decisions you made as a young child. You will recognize a positive habit - it vitalizes, invigorates and motivates you - it may even inspire you! IMPORTANT* REMEMBER THAT YOUR HABITS SHOULD BE THE RESULT OF A CONSCIOUS CHOICE!

» Repeat this affirmation:

I AM AWARE OF ALL MY HABITS SO AS TO REALIZE WHICH ARE OF BENEFIT TO ME IN MY DEVELOPMENT AND ARE CONTRIBUTING TO MY HARMONY. I ACCEPT THAT LIFE IS A CHOICE I HAVE MADE.

CHAPTER 15

THE EGO

"Ego", or false pride, is an uncomfortable subject for most people to discuss. All of these stem from fear - and so we are face to face with fear that we have tried our whole lives to cover up with ego. Although aware of our Divine Perfection subconsciously, we have yet to understand the need to surrender to its simplicity and guidance. We still need to "control". I have yet to meet a person who has completely mastered his ego, although every religion honors someone who has.

Those with strong egos are easily identified - they continually seek to be "right", blaming, criticizing and judging others, trying to change them to feel superior. Power over others, which is only an illusion, gives them strength that they are lacking inwardly. The more egotistical a person seems outwardly, the more fear he is dealing with inside. Mankind's ego is its greatest downfall - it is the root cause of rivalries between individuals and nations, wars, intrigue and hatred. It breeds a shallow, empty power but hardens the heart and prevents love. Ego-driven people deem themselves "winners", but are, in truth, the real losers.

By allowing your ego to overtake you, you stand to lose many things. The repercussions in your relationships, your health and your happiness are severe. You will perceive life as a constant "fight", an uphill battle. Is it worth it?

Egotistical people are infatuated with themselves - their personas. They are completely out of touch with themselves, so any attempt to enlighten them is futile and will be met with contempt. They have no tolerance for the opinions of others -especially concerning themselves, if they do not coincide with theirs. They prefer the company of those who gratify them. Good deeds are done only with ulterior motives and with a secret desire to be applauded and glorified. Many otherwise balanced people who start something with pure intentions, find that things turn sour when poisoned by the ego. Be aware, and beware, of both forms of false pride - intellectual and spiritual pride.

INTELLECTUAL PRIDE is characterized by know-it-all behavior, such as lack of tolerance of others' opinions and interruption when others are speaking. This type of person talks loudly and quickly and will do whatever it takes to maintain the undivided attention of those around him until he finally has them in his grasp and they say "Oh, yes, we understand and agree with you"...so, he must be right!

Another typical trait of this personality type is the frequent use of the phrase "I knew it!" How often do you find yourself saying this? Be careful. It indicates a need to have your ego stroked. A person who really knew everything would not feel compelled to say so. Knowledge is a deeply private thing to be shared only when one is asked to do so - when another person opens that door. Forcing the door open is an ego trip.

Ego resists all inner transformation and blinds you from seeing God in everytHing and everyone. It represses feelings and emotions and denies relationship with the true self. It will discourage you from self-improvement and will not allow you to forgive, lest you are perceived as "admitting you were wrong!"

The purpose of the existence of the ego is to challenge you to overcome its illusion. When you are overwhelmed with ego, you are no longer yourself. The ego is the thorn that constantly irritates and keeps you aware that there is still more growing to do - as long as you continue to feel the thorn, you will be aware of the need to move away from it. Acknowledge it - give it a name if you wish. Whenever you are aware of its irritating presence, tell it that you no longer have any need for it. By doing so, you will have great impact on its disappearance and will no longer be under its influence.

Keep in mind that your ego is stubborn and will do whatever it takes in order to survive. It doesn't like to be mastered, as it perceives itself as the master. It will torment and attack you once you decide to do without it, especially the first few weeks following your decision to do so. In my own experience, it takes approximately three weeks for the ego's resistance to subside and for things to get easier.

Your ego is frightened. It can be compared to a neighbor who comes over any time of night or day to tell you his horror stories - and you let him continue to do so. Once you have had enough and tell him "Get out- I don't want to listen anymore", he will be angered and offended. He has lost ground with you and will attempt several times to regain it. You must stay alert to maintain your position and your power over it.

The ego is very prominent and has ruled the behavior of mankind for centuries. Ego is the exaltation of our lower self, which represents your personality opposed to the "I", which represents your higher self, or your individuality. As you develop your individuality or higher self, the ego will lose its grip on you. It will not be mastered easily, but through consistent, gentle, simple acts of love on a daily basis, the ego will be tamed.

SPIRITUAL PRIDE is characterized by a "Holier than thou" attitude and is often exhibited by people who have embarked on their journeys of personal development. They have not let go of their egos yet and, having discovered what they feel as the "right" path, they feel superior to those who have not. " They are not as enlightened as I am" is often a thought that crosses the minds of those who have begun to grow. Beware of this pride, this sense of superiority, as it is false. It will undermine the very development you are now enjoying.

Remain alert as your consciousness unfolds. Your value as a human being is neither more nor less than that of any other being, regardless of your level of development. All souls are pure - only their expression varies. An elevated state is not a superior state.

It would be absurd to say an elephant had more value than a mouse, for example - for each is a manifestation of God.

A person who displays his ego, attracts other egos that are, by nature, confrontational. This is a good lesson in mastering the ego: When you are with someone who is determined to have the last word, do not insist on having yours. Accept that he is clinging to an important belief, which is his truth, and accept that HE MAY BE RIGHT! You are probably both right!

Therefore, deep down, as you accept that the other is right, you come in touch with your own truth. Here is what I suggest you say: "I accept that, for you, it is a very important point of view", even if you don't understand it. The other person will be completely stunned.

An egotistical person always wants to win and to have the impression that the other has "lost", or submitted to him. With the phrase I have given you, he feels he has been accepted without his having to feel superior. In this way, you have not submitted to him, but have neutralized any conflict and created a common ground of balance and harmony that even his ego (and yours) will be comfortable with.

If you were to change your views for the sole purpose of agreeing with someone else, you have submitted to him. You both lose - you, having submitted, have lost your power and depleted your energy; he has lost by accepting the illusion of power, of winning, that was stolen from others, rather than having been drawn from his inner self. Anyone who uses his ego to win over others is a loser.

The opposite of ego is humility. Be careful, though, many people who consider themselves humble are actually exhibiting a false humility that masks fear and weakness causing them to give up easily. Give these people some power and a false pride rapidly emerges, replacing their "humility". Those who cannot accept compliments, who put themselves down in terms of their talents and abilities, are acting from false humility, which is another form of ego. The true self is fully aware of its talents and abilities and it neither needs to hide them nor to blatantly expose them. It accepts them and nurtures them; it also feels no pride in them and no guilt for having them.

If you must compare yourself with someone else whom you feel is superior to you in any way, do so by understanding that God's presence is in all of us and that person is expressing his God-self more effectively than you. You will understand that there is always much to be learned from others.

Ego breeds hypocrisy, vanity and the lust for power. There are two types of hypocrisy- the one of the great man who pretends to be ordinary and the ordinary man who pretends to be great. The first exhibits false humility, the other, false pride.

If only egotistical people knew what awaited them after death, what they will have to experience between lives and what they are creating for their next life! Although discussions of the spiritual realm are not the purpose of this book, I will touch on the importance of mastery of the ego. It is vital that you become conscious of what motivates you. Is it to be glorified and flattered by others, or is it the importance of being "right"? Take a good look at what it is costing you. The consequences will be carried with you on your soul's journey into the next world and beyond.

Do you help others in order to be recognized and applauded? Do you want everyone to know what wonderful things you are doing for others? Take a good look at yourself! If someone you were helping was ungrateful to you and did not acknowledge your contribution to his success, would you be disappointed? If he had experienced some major transformation in his life, with your help, and did not acknowledge you, would you feel he "owed" you something? That is your ego wanting to be recognized.

Reading this may disturb you, as you are beginning to realize how much control your ego has over you. Become conscious of that. Keeping your ego fed is taking food away from your own soul. A well-fed ego results in a soul that is starving. Which is more important to you?

A strong, fully grown ego has sucked all the love out of your heart, causing "hardening of the heart". This condition can be reversed by allowing love to flow through the heart , washing over it and dissolving the ego, until the heart is revived and fully-functioning again. You and everyone around you will be brought back to life. The ego is like a cancer of the heart, feeding on it and destroying the love and peace that reside there. Let the love pour out and the life flow.

Use your mind to uplift, not to put down. Simple, sincere acts of love and kindness last so much longer than being "right" in the eyes of others - and they run much deeper. Forget the shallow, empty satisfaction that the ego seeks.

You may be aware of ties with your parents that have not been cut; your ego causes you to hesitate in addressing these ties. It tells you not to "give in" or admit defeat. Asking their forgiveness, or offering an act of love, does not mean you have won or lost! Accept that you both have done your best according to your level of awareness and did not properly express love at the time. Take the first step now - do it from the heart; let go of your ego. Have that heart-to-heart talk and feel the love and acceptance pour out and wash over both of you.

Each simple act of LOVE heals and transforms. Love is the ultimate healing power - it brings about physical, mental, emotional and spiritual healing.

By now, it must be very clear to you that the ego is forged from fear - fear of being unloved, rejected, judged or criticized, fear of not living up to expectations (thereby losing something or someone that matters to you). When you find yourself in the company of an egotistical person, try to feel the fear and suffering that underlies his behavior. He may try to change you or frighten you by forcing his overbearing and uncompromising attitude on you. Don't be impressed - he is more insecure than you are. Don't respond to him with your mind, but touch him with your heart.

CHAPTER 15 EXERCISES

» Make a list of the people you have come into contact with over the past three days. You may have met with them, spoken with them, or merely thought of them.

» Be totally honest with yourself. No one else will see what you are writing. If you like, you can burn the paper when you are done. With each contact, ask yourself whether your ego got the better of you - did your intellectual pride tell you "I knew best" or your spiritual pride tell you "I am better"?

» The point of this exercise is not to stir up guilt, but to raise your consciousness and clarify your position in respect to your ego. What did these responses, and your overall attitude, cost you in terms of your inner peace, your social life, happiness and attitude toward others? Are you prepared to continue paying that price?

» Confront your ego directly and observe the changes in your life. They will be dramatic.

» Take each incident on your list, one at a time, and discuss it openly with the person involved. Ask for forgiveness, if you need to, and tell them that you realize it was your ego talking and not your heart. Admit, simply, that you are a 'WORK IN PROGRESS' and ask for their patience. That beautiful act of love will have tremendous significance in your growth...and theirs.

» Here is your affirmation. Repeat it as often as you can:

I ACCEPT MYSELF AS I AM, EACH DAY
LEARNING TO MASTER MY EGO BY SEEING
AND FEELING GOD IN EVERYONE AND
EVERYTHING AROUND ME.

CHAPTER 16

FALSE MASTERS

In this chapter I will touch on and briefly discuss some of the most common false masters. Firstly, you must understand fully that there is only ONE TRUE MASTER, and that is your inner God - your God-self. Every human being has his own, individual master within.

Webster's defines "Master" as " One with control or authority over another". Many people find that their lives are ruled, or run, by others (e.i.. spouse, children, parents, authority figures, etc.), a situation that is the result of fear. In my workshops, I have made the following observation on many occasions:

In the past, I gave evening sessions and some of the women in my workshop often became nervous and impatient around 10:30 p.m. because the sessions usually ended at that time. If the class ran a little longer, they began to feel uneasy, knowing that they would have to deal with their spouse waiting for them. They would begin to get restless on their chairs and often get up to check through the window. As soon as their mate would arrive, they would leave and miss the end of the session. A woman who acts this way fears her mate. She is afraid of displeasing him. Rather than put herself (and him) in an uncomfortable situation, she should arrange for him to arrive a little later , or make alternate arrangements for transportation.

When you fear someone else, you are allowing him to become your master...and you are no longer your own master. He will manipulate you constantly, as he knows exactly what triggers a reaction in you. Being in a reactive state is very draining on your energy and creates a chronic emotional state that is detrimental to your physical, mental, and spiritual health.

THE NEWS, surprisingly enough, is another false master. Remember that the news and weather reports are MEDIA-GENER-

ATED! They are carefully designed to hold your interest. Whether listening to the radio, reading the newspaper or watching television, people often base their daily decisions on the weather forecast; if inclement weather is expected, they will change their plans, yet the forecasts are often inaccurate! Did you know that human beings have an influence on the outside temperature? In a given geographic area, if the majority of people suddenly were to change their thoughts from sadness to happiness (rain or sunshine), the temperature would change accordingly. Remember that the earth is a living entity whose cells are closely tied with our own - they respond accordingly.

Someone who is easily influenced by the news will live in fear most of the time. "Good" news is not "interesting" news, so that what we hear and see is usually something negative. If there is news on a particular day about financial problems in the country, some people will hide their money or transfer it to another country. If we hear about a young boy found mutilated by his aggressor, we can become emotionally involved and affected for days. It is important to remain detached from the experiences of others and to accept that we are not responsible for the lives of others. We will then be able to feel compassion without torment.

POWER AND RECOGNITION are always false masters. As discussed in the last chapter, "Ego", these are characteristics of false pride and the need for them is generated by the appetite of the ego. Doing something for the purpose of gaining recognition and/or power indicates that you are a slave to outside influence and not in control of your inner self. You are out of touch with your God-self and your true nature.

MATERIAL POSSESSIONS are often false masters. Take a good look at how you feel about your own belongings. Do you treasure them? If your favorite possession was lost or damaged, how would you react...with anger? If the answer is yes, your material possessions are in control of you. What difference will it make in your next life if you die short of one crystal glass, or if there is a small scratch on your dining room table...or a spot on the rug? Put these things in perspective.

It is normal and healthy to want to be surrounded by beautiful things. Our environment is important to us. What is not beneficial, though, is to let material possessions rule your life. They are there to embellish your life, not to govern it.

ASTROLOGY can also become a false master, if used to guide your every decision. Many people have their astral charts done and follow them closely, determining every decision based on the position of the planets. The astral chart is only a tool to help you become aware of your astral influences; what governs your life are the decisions you make and the actions you take. You chose your astral sign solely for the purpose of learning to evolve and love in spite of various astral influences. Once you understand these influences, you will master them.

Consider this situation as an analogy to the astral connection: For a year you are assigned to a post with a very negative person. You are not given a choice; you have to work closely for a one-year period. If you are conscious of the negative influence, you will remain alert and be in a better position to deal with it. The same applies to your astral position: although you are prone to specific influence, your decisions are your own.

CLAIRVOYANTS AND MEDIUMS become false masters for a growing number of people. As our collective awareness increases, more clairvoyants are emerging. What actually happens when you consult a psychic? Psychics, also known as "sensitives", or "channels", pick up on the vibrations of your subtle bodies. They are in tune with your current state of mind and current state of affairs as they relate to your vibration. They are able to tell you what will happen if you remain on the path you are on. As the future is entirely dependent on the choices you make right now, the clairvoyant is able to "predict" your future based on your current vibration. If, for whatever reason, you alter your frame of mind in the near future, you will be redirecting your life accordingly. The predictions will then no longer apply. If, however, you allow psychics to have enough influence on you, you will continue in the same vein and their predictions will "come true". REMEMBER: Only you determine your future and it is created entirely through your own thoughts and your decisions.

You can continuously change your path during the course of your life; you can also go through several lifetimes at once, if you choose to. A radical change will give you the feeling that you have been "reborn" and you will feel like a new person. Those around you will be amazed by your transformation and will exclaim: "My God, we don't recognize you anymore! What have you done to yourself...you're not even the same person!" Such pronounced transformation occurs when you have made a change in your mainstream. This type of rapid evolution reduces the number of times you will have to return to the earth plane - it accelerates your spiritual development.

ORGANIZED RELIGIONS that proclaim they alone are in sole possession of the truth and you, therefore, must adhere to their rules, have exposed themselves as powerful false masters. If your life is being ruled by a religion, cult or sect with its own notion of right and wrong, you are no longer master of your own life. Religions were organized centuries ago to establish a framework of behaviors for cultures that were not conscious enough to guide themselves. As with everything, there are positive and negative aspects to any religion that has developed for such purposes. Many of the religions, because they are created by human beings, are designed to control their followers by instilling fear in them. This is a terrible abuse of power and does not result in the balanced, harmonious existence that you desire. God is love - the concept of fear is man-made. If your religion is causing you to feel fear of any kind, understand that it is inappropriate and detrimental to your spiritual growth.

Today's religions are more in alignment with the concept of love. Once you become more in tune with your inner knowing, you will understand what you need and will gravitate to a religion that is comfortable and beneficial to you.

DOCTORS sometimes fall into the 'false master' category. Once you learn to trust your inner master, you will find you have no need to continually consult your physician before making many of the decisions in your life (i.e.: whether or not to take a vacation, move, change careers, etc.) For example, a patient who is considering a career move, but feels nervous and apprehensive about it, may be advised by his doctor to avoid making such a move. This patient would be wise to look inside himself, determine what is causing his fear and then listen to what his body is telling him. He will then become his own master.

There has been a powerful movement toward holistic medicine in the past few years , based on an understanding of the correlation between the mind and the body and a focus on the prevention of disease. Once you learn to listen to your body, you will become attuned to its signals and its needs and will begin to enjoy a health and wholeness that are the natural state. Hand-in-hand, you and your body will take control of your health.

MEDICATION becomes another false master, once you have relinquished control of your health. There is a pill for everything - for headaches, backaches, bellyaches, for sleeping, for waking, to calm you or to give you more energy, for breathing, digesting, assimilating, eliminating...whatever you can imagine, there's a pill for it! EVERY MEDICATION HAS SIDE EFFECTS, which is your body's way of rebelling. If you think that medication is transforming you, you are right...to the detriment of your health and well-being. Decide to use medication only when you have reached your limits and you really need it. Take control and become your own master!

ILLNESS is a false master to those who accept that sickness is normal. It is not. The natural state of the body is healthy.

FASHION is one of the most ludicrous false masters, governing the lives of those who live in fear of what others will think of them.

WORK, if it becomes an obsession, is a false master. For those whose identities are determined by their work, the thought of relaxing, or not working for any period of time, causes tremendous discomfort. They can't let go of it long enough to enjoy their families, to take a vacation, or just to smell the flowers. No one, on their deathbed, ever said: "I wish I had spent more time at the office..." Ask yourself if your work is fulfilling to you. Does it help you to uplift others? Does it give you a sense of peace and satisfaction? If your work allows you to grow, spiritually, you are on the right track. If you are working strictly for the money, the power or the recognition, you are no longer in control. It has become your master.

SUPERSTITION can become a false master, if taken seriously and used to determine choices in your life, or even in determining the direction of your day.

EGO, FEAR & GUILT are powerful false masters in that they govern decisions based on reactive behavior stemming from emotional, irrational thinking. Refer to Chapter fifteen for information on ego and to Chapter nineteen for guilt and fear.

MONEY is probably the most prevalent false master in our materialistic culture. It rules, or at least has some bearing on, nearly every decision people make. Again, like all false masters, the preoccupation with money and the resulting control it has over a person's life, stems from insecurity and fear of being without. Ask yourself if your bank account determines most of your daily decisions. Is it limiting you in any way from getting what you want? It's time to adjust your attitude about money, so that you fully understand that it is energy to be tapped at will.

Just like electricity, water and wind, money is a form of energy that exists in abundance. Like all energies, it has power and is there for the taking. Accumulating it out of fear of not having enough, and hanging on to it, are indications of lack of faith or confidence in Divine Law.

Compare money to sunshine. Whether there are 3 or 300 people sunbathing on a beach will have no bearing on the amount of sunlight being generated. It is very important for you to understand that money is a form of energy - the more you allow it to circulate, the more it will flow into your life, gain power, momentum and multiply.

The same holds true for many things. Each corn or tomato seed, properly planted, will produce dozens of other tomatoes or ears of corn. If not properly sowed and nurtured, or if kept in a drawer, those seeds will not be brought to life.

Letting go of financial insecurity can be a long process if you fail to understand its energy. Take a look back in your life. If there was something you desired a great deal, did you not find the money to buy it somehow? Did you suffer terribly having channeled that money into something you really wanted? I would venture a guess that you bought it and that it brought joy to you, enhancing your life and feeding your energy. YOU ARE WORTH IT!

The image you have of yourself - your sense of SELF-WORTH is determined by you and you alone. Others mirror whatever opinion you have of yourself. If you prefer to keep money in case of bad luck, you will attract bad luck. If you prefer, instead, to honor yourself by taking a vacation, you will appreciate what money can really do for your inner self. You will always manage, somehow, to make ends meet.

When shopping for groceries, be aware of your mindset. Is it "the price" that determines what you are eating? I'm not suggesting that you avoid items that are "on special" - buying something you wanted in the first place, at a better price, is simply a wise thing to do. If, however, you buy something of lesser quality, or a brand you would prefer not to buy, just because it is cheaper, you are short-changing yourself and giving yourself the wrong message. Tell yourself you are worthy of the best and you will have it!

Start with small daily victories - keep your bearings and don't overextend yourself. For example, don't start with the mansion on the beach, or the Mercedes just yet, but buy yourself top-quality produce instead of the bruised, half-price produce. Begin to increase your vibration by realizing your own worth. You will then begin to reap accordingly, as you get into the flow of energy that money generates. The more you let it circulate, the more you will receive. Be careful that your new sense of self-worth comes from your true self and not from your ego-self. If it comes from your ego-self, you will still be seeking self-gratification and the mindset will be all wrong. Instead, surrender to the flow and enjoy.

Let go of the fear; put your "in case of" aside and go on that vacation. Forget asking yourself "what if.........happens?"

If it happens, know that you are capable of dealing with it. You will manage to make ends meet and still enjoy your life, if you have faith.

If you decide you really want something, you will make it happen! Most people put their priorities in the wrong place. If they are told their television set is too old and not worth repairing, they run out and buy another one. Somehow, they will find the means to pay for it. How necessary is a television set? Yet, if you determine that you REALLY NEED one, you will manage to get one.

Some of the people who are interested in taking classes at my Center balk at the price when it is presented to them. The same people spend thousands of dollars to help others, or to buy material things, but do not deem themselves worthy enough to spend a few hundred dollars on their own transformation and inner happiness! When you buy a gift for someone else, do you find that you often get them something you would like to receive yourself? Treat yourself that way - you are your best friend!

Observe the influence money has on your life. As long as it is your master, you will be stifled. Once you have mastered it and understood it, the changes in your life will be profound!

If you believe in the great law "You reap what you sow", here's a little secret: start right now to send thoughts of prosperity to everyone you know. Wish them as much money as they want. The energy will circulate to such a degree that you will find it comes back to you much more quickly than it would have if you'd only been thinking about your own prosperity.

As you know by now, you are not here to change everyone around you - you are here to transform your own frame of mind. Put your new thoughts and ideas into practice and it will begin to manifest all around you. Do not let the opinions and criticisms of others undermine what you are doing.

If you have decided to adopt a positive attitude toward money and wish to master it, you will understand that it is a private journey to be taken on your own. Others will change when they are ready - to each his own evolution. Once you have achieved happiness and inner peace, others will feel it, as you radiate it.

Once you have mastered money, you will always have enough. Your savings will no longer be motivated by fear; only your surplus funds will be set aside.

CHAPTER 16 EXERCISES

» Make a list of all the false masters you can identify in your own life.

» Determine which of the false masters you have identified is the one that influences you the most. For the next three days, resolve to remain aware of this false master and to take back control. Do not go on to the next chapter without having done this exercise.

» Your level of awareness of the false masters in your life will determine the speed of your personal development! Once you have learned to overcome your false masters, you will truly begin to master your own life.

» Here is your affirmation. Repeat it often through the next three days:

I AM THE SOLE MASTER OF MY LIFE.
I REALIZE THAT I CREATE WITH MY OWN

THOUGHTS. I BECOME WHAT I THINK; MY HAPPINESS, PROSPERITY, LOVE AND HARMONY ARE DEPENDENT ON MY THOUGHTS.

CHAPTER 17

MENTAL ESSENTIALS

There are many fundamental needs of the mental body, a few of which I will discuss in this chapter. Failure to meet any one of these needs will have a negative impact on your physical, mental, emotional and, especially, your spiritual life.

TRUTH is the most important need. It is the key to freedom, uplifting your higher body and expanding your vibration. Your superconscious mind reacts to lies as a violation of the inner self, whether the lies come from someone else or from yourself. You will experience an unpleasant feeling when faced with a lie. To say "it does not bother me" is an indication that you feel the opposite. It does bother you; covering up that discomfort will not make it go away.

To be "true" means that what you think, say and do are the same thing. When your words and actions do not coincide with your thoughts, you are out of alignment and your inner balance will be off. If someone asks you your opinion, you owe it to yourself to be truthful, for the sake of your own alignment, if nothing else.

JUSTICE is an element of the truth. Note the discomfort that an act of injustice against you, or against anyone else causes you. Perhaps you have witnessed a mother acting unjustly toward her child (perhaps his needs come last, for example). Instinctively you feel compassion for the child. Acting unjustly toward yourself creates the same inner conflict. Your superconscious mind, your soul, needs to be nurtured and kept whole. Any behavior or attitude that is contrary to that wholeness is unhealthy. The body provides signals to the person who is not true or unjust to himself, by affecting the throat region and/or the respiratory system.

INDIVIDUALITY, as defined by Webster, is "the aggregate of characteristics that distinguishes one person from others". You are unique and must respect and express that uniqueness to be true to yourself. Stop concerning yourself with the opinions others have of you, or with their expectations of you - BE YOURSELF. Teenagers are caught up in the struggle of "finding themselves". It is a critical phase and, often, a painful one, as they are trying hard to express themselves and need more space than most people in which to spread their wings. They easily feel smothered by parents and others who try to cast them in molds that do not fit. Keep in mind, when raising your own adolescents, that the mold you are trying to cram them into may be one that you didn't have the nerve to fit into yourself.

Children of the New Age are much more in tune with Natural Laws and sensitive to individual expression of their true nature. If they are not allowed to express themselves, they may experience allergies and respiratory problems.

RESPECT of ourselves and others is vital to our mental health and balance. It is terribly frustrating to have to respect someone of authority (i.e.: police, teachers, employers, parents, etc.) when the respect is not mutual. A position of authority does not give one a license to disrespect and abuse others. No one is superior to another on a soul level. A desire to change another person in any way, shape or form indicates a lack of respect for them. If others do not respect you, remember that they are mirroring your own opinion toward them.

Acknowledge the importance of Truth, Justice, Individuality and Respect as necessities in the maintenance of your overall health. Just as air is important to the survival of your physical body, so are these essential to the survival of your mental body.

SECURITY, in the true sense of the word, is the peace of mind created by the thought that there is nothing to fear, therefore, security lies in the absence of fear. Understanding this creates peace of mind, which is the ultimate outcome of security. Many people misinterpret security as having a good savings account "to fall back on", or a job with a good benefits package "just in case...", or a good stock of material possessions, or even a spouse. Real security is knowing that, no matter what happens, you have what you need inside of you to make your life work and to get the results you want. Depending on anything outside of you to provide for you, should make you feel insecure, because, ultimately, you are giving away your power. *The only true security is within you.*

Feelings of insecurity manifest themselves in the physical body as lower back and lower abdominal discomfort. Fear of the future affects the legs and preoccupation with money affects the sciatic nerve (a signal from the body that your fear of financial inadequacy is not well-founded). You may notice that insecure people frequently chew on the inside of their mouths.

INTEGRITY, according to Webster, means "personal honesty and independence". It also means completeness and unity. Integrity is derived from the word "Integration", in other words, "as without, so within". You say what you mean in your heart. There is no "hidden agenda", no "reading between the lines". Someone who does not keep his word or does not honor his engagements, promises or duties, is being dishonest with others and, especially, with himself. This type of person will find his dishonesty manifests physically through digestive problems (i.e.: indigestion, diarrhea and liver malfunction). A person who carries guilt resulting from dishonest behavior, may bring about an accident.

Bad breath is often caused by shameful, though unconscious, thoughts that a person does not want to reveal to anyone. This person considers himself "dirty" inside. His bad breath is a signal from his supserconscious mind to "clean up his act".

GUIDANCE refers to the need to be of service to others. It is a return to Divine Perfection. Although we feel a need to help and guide others, we often go about it the wrong way by giving advice and making decisions for others. To guide is to share knowledge without expectations. It is up to the other person to determine whether or not he will accept and utilize this knowledge. Be sure to share your knowledge only when the door is open for the other person to receive it. Unsolicited advice is unwelcome and untimely.

If you feel a strong need to share your knowledge with someone, be certain that he wants to receive it. If he does not, keep it to yourself and accept that he is not in a position to receive or to benefit from it at that particular time. If he accepts your advice, give it freely without expectation or stipulation. He will do what he wants with it according to his own needs and his own time frame. It is your gift to him. Remember expectations come from your own ego - from its need to be gratified.

Feelings of unworthiness, or feeling like neither you nor your advice is welcome, will be manifested on the physical level as elimination problems of the kidneys or intestines. Arthritis is often the result of feeling "taken advantage of" and is usually experienced by someone who feels a need to give advice to others , with expectations of "a return on his investment of time and energy". In this case, the "help" is given with strings attached. Not having these expectations met leaves one feeling lonely and worthless.

A SENSE OF PURPOSE, or a "reason for being" is vital. It provides enthusiasm and energy that propels you through your day. Are you proud of what you do for a living? Do you get excited when you talk about your work and do you feel you have a reason for being on the planet? You have to feed your soul; to be creative and to tap into the pool of energy that is your very life-force. Without doing so, you will experience lethargy and anemia - so get your blood flowing and bring yourself to life! If you are not sure what gets you really motivated, find out and DO IT!

CHAPTER 17 EXERCISES

» Write down the needs of the mental body and examine the ones you have neglected in your own life. In doing so, you will begin to understand the underlying dissatisfaction you feel. It is up to you to nourish your mental body. There is no way around it - these needs must be met, as they are necessary for your survival and your overall health.

» Determine to address each of these needs and take action. Only in doing so will you get closer to obtaining your dreams.

» Repeat this affirmation daily:

I AM NOW DETERMINED TO RESPECT THE NEEDS OF MY MENTAL BODY AND THEREFORE REGAIN MY MENTAL BALANCE.

PART FOUR:

LISTEN TO YOUR EMOTIONAL BODY

CHAPTER 18

EMOTIONAL EXPRESSION

If you've come this far in the book and done the exercises, you've undoubtedly gone through some emotional upheaval. Hopefully, this chapter will help you to understand and express some of the emotions you've been experiencing.

Webster defines emotion simply as "a strong feeling". These "feelings" include sadness, happiness, fear, empathy, jealousy, regret, hatred, anger, elation, joy and many more. Improperly identifying or expressing any one of them brings about frustration, confusion and agitation. All emotions are the result of reaction to outside stimulus. They are all brought on by fear. Negative emotions drain your energy by lowering the vibration of your magnetic field. Positive emotions increase that field, through the bonding and merging that occurs in synergy with other positive fields. That is why love heals and hatred destroys to the degree the emotion is felt.

What does it mean to "express" an emotion? Many people in my workshops have come to me and said: "I have been in therapy for many years and I am constantly told that I need to express my emotions, but no one can tell me how to do it. Do I need to cry and scream and break dishes? What do I do?"

I have developed an effective method that will enable you to express your emotions without causing any damage to those people or possessions around you. It is simple and effective. Understand that you will be unable to master any emotion that cannot be expressed.

The same external stimulus will continue to test you until you no longer react. Take, for example, a husband who has gotten into the habit of humiliating his wife in front of his family. something displeases him, he makes a point of waiting until the family is around to tell her about it. She is angry inside, wondering why he cannot discuss it with her privately. She will continue to be angry unless she addresses it.

How many emotional situations have recurred in your life since your childhood because you were not equipped to express yourself correctly? Meanwhile, your emotions are repressed and some of the following common behaviors are engaged in to pacify yourself: eating or drinking for emotional comfort, taking medication to calm yourself, sitting in front of the television set to distract yourself (or seeing a movie, sleeping or reading for the same reason), or taking a warm bath to relax, etc.

When you are angry, it is not of any benefit to pretend you are not. Some people sit and think about it, waiting for "just the right time" to clear the situation up, others smoke or drink, cry, work, do housework, handiwork, or simply refuse to talk. All of these behaviors are meant to distract you or help you ignore what you are feeling. Some people take a more active approach by engaging in a violent sport or choosing to become malicious directly or indirectly toward the other person. Pretending it doesn't bother you is a critical mistake.

Another very common reaction is to "dump" on a third party. For example: the husband, having a bad day at work, comes home and "dumps" it all on his wife. This is not beneficial to any relationship! The husband who subjects his wife to this, does so with expectations that he will be told he is "right" and be comforted and gratified. After she does so, he feels satisfied, saying: "Ah, talking to you helps me so much! You always find the right thing to say!" But has anything been resolved? No - she has just allowed her energy to be drained. As months and years go by, she will feel more and more depleted until their relationship is undermined. He will feel less and less gratified as she is less able to give him her energy. The same thing often happens between friends. The "dumper" is only temporarily boosted and will need another "fix" the next day. The "dumpee" has nothing to gain, as he allows his energy to be continually fed upon.

There is a solution. If you are the dumpee, listen patiently to the dumper, then say to him: "What do you intend to do to solve your problem?" Most likely he will reply: "What do you expect me to do? It is their fault - there is nothing I can do." Then you gently tell that person that you are no longer interested in listening to his problems because he obviously enjoys having them and giving them power. He sustains them by continually focusing on them and amplifying them. You will no longer allow him to feed your energy to his problems.

He may be shocked, find you unfair, uncaring and harsh; but he may be shocked enough to realize that there is truth in what you have just said to him. If he was merely using you as his dumping ground, he will find someone else to dump on and you will have not lost anything. You will, however, have managed to hang onto your energy. To discuss your problems for the sole purpose of feeling better afterward is called "dumping". To share something, on the other hand, even something unpleasant, with the intention of finding a solution or bringing about change, is a healthy process. In "sharing", you have no expectations of the other person and are not handing your responsibility over to them. That is why it is important for spouses to learn to share their positive and negative experiences the way two good friends would do it.

To properly express and deal with an emotion, identify it and be objective about it. Say: "Yes, I am angry. This is what I am angry about - can you help me find a solution?" The worst thing you can do is repress or ignore what you are feeling, pretending that it has no effect on you.

People often say: "I will not give him the satisfaction of letting him know I am angry." Remember - repressed emotions are often manifested as obesity and disease. UNEXPRESSED EMOTIONS SIT IN THE CELLS OF THE BODY AND ALTER THE BODY CHEMISTRY.

Releasing your emotions through crying, walking or getting involved in sports is better than repressing them, but will not address their cause. You will continue to react to whatever stimulates that particular emotion in you until you resolve and dissolve what is triggering it.

Here are the steps that I suggest you take in order to come to terms with your emotions. Take these steps one at a time, with sincerity, and you will find that you remain detached in the face of whatever outside stimulus you reacted to previously. You will be able to acknowledge the situation as it reoccurs, but will be free from the emotional response. You will finally be free from the emotional bondage that has kept you hostage, possibly since childhood, if you address them one at a time!

STEP ONE: Identify the emotion. It is important to know EXACTLY what you are feeling - is it anger, disappointment, frustration, sadness, fear, anxiety, aggression, hatred...? Some of these feel quite similar. Identify it clearly. Note that two or more emotions can surface simultaneously.

STEP TWO: Accept RESPONSIBILITY for your response. Understand completely that you have chosen to feel this particular emotion. No on "made you feel this way". You have allowed yourself to be affected by an external factor. To take responsibility for your emotion may be difficult to do in the heat of the moment, initially, but it is a critical step. Mostly, it is the ego that is having the difficulty. In order to do so, you will have to learn to step back and be objective about what you are feeling.

Here's an example: A close friend of yours approaches you, wearing a new dress. You can't help noticing that the color of the dress doesn't suit her at all - that it seems to drain the color from her face, leaving her looking lifeless and much older. You say to yourself: "Gee, I should really say something - someone has to tell her so that she doesn't embarrass herself by wearing that again!" So, you take it upon yourself to be the one to do her that favor.

Your friend can then choose one of the following reactions:

1."Oh, thanks for telling me! I've never worn this color before. I wasn't sure how it would look on me. It must have taken a lot of courage for you to say something. I appreciate it!" She is grateful that you shared your opinion.

2."I don't really care what you think - I like it." No fuss, no emotion. She remains neutral and unaffected.

3."I didn't ask for your opinion! Who do you think you are? I don't give a damn what you think of my dress!" Inwardly, she is plotting her revenge.

Take a close look at the third possible response. Whether or not she actually expresses her anger, what really caused it? Her reaction indicates that she is uncomfortable being perceived as "unacceptable". It is her ego that has been bruised.

All emotions stem from the same source - the mind. They are NEVER CAUSED BY SOMEONE ELSE! NEVER! YOU ARE SOLELY RESPONSIBLE FOR YOUR EMOTIONS!

Return to the example of the husband who humiliates his wife in front of his family. She would not feel anger if she took responsibility for her emotions. She would feel compassion for him, thinking: "Poor man, he must be afraid of me if he cannot talk about it when we are alone together. What attitude do I have toward him that scares him to the point of not revealing his opinions to me? Am I too authoritarian with him? Do I really listen when he gives me his opinion or do I hurry to convince him of mine?"

Once you understand that you always reap what you sow, you will have a different attitude about a given situation. If, for example, you experience a similar situation in your own life, accept your responsibility, rather than allowing his attitude to upset you. You may begin to realize that you, too, are very critical of him, even in his absence. You probably would like to change him - he can feel that, even if you have never expressed it and he is "taking control" by humiliating you. It is his way of claiming his space. He feels, unconsciously, that you have stifled him and resorts automatically to his basic instinct of self-preservation. Whenever he pushes your buttons, causing you to react, he is trying to tell you that you have been encroaching on his territory.

By accepting responsibility for your reaction, your emotions will dissipate. The anger you feel toward him will diminish as you begin to understand what he is feeling.

STEP THREE: Express yourself clearly and concisely to the person concerned. You may not feel this step is necessary if you have accepted full responsibility with all your heart, but I suggest that you attempt it anyway. Once you are secure in accepting full responsibility for your reaction, you have nothing to lose by discussing the occurrence with the person concerned. This will confirm that you have understood your responsibility with the heart and not with the mind.

Using the same example, you may want to express yourself in the following manner:

Arriving home with your husband after another of these incidents, you explain that you are angry and why. Tell him also that, after a great deal of reflection, you realize that you've been infringing on his space by being critical or demanding of him. Tell him that you now understand that his behavior is his way of putting you "in your place" (and out of his space). You had not seen things in that light before.

Be sure to express yourself AFTER you have accepted your responsibility. If you try to do so without clearly accepting full responsibility first, any residual blame you may be feeling will be very apparent. Expressing yourself prematurely will still generate accusation on your part. If you say: "I'll try not to let your behavior bother me - I'm sure you have your reasons.", you have not come far enough. He will still hear that it is his fault. If only he would change, you would be happier. That's what he will make of your exchange. The more you try to change him, the more he will resist and the more often the situation will reoccur. CHANGE YOURSELF and accept responsibility for your reaction.

To my knowledge, the most efficient way to change a situation like this is to follow your heart. Before discussing it with him, be sure you have completed the process of accepting that only you, with your attitude, have created it, or allowed it to continue. You reap what you sow. With daily practice, you will learn to accept responsibility for what happens around you and be able to diffuse any situation that previously caused you to react emotionally.

Emotional Mastery requires commitment and perseverance. I don't know of anyone who has completely overcome this problem. Try to imagine a friend of yours coming to you and saying: "You said or did something that really hurt me (or made me angry, or whatever), but I realize now that I didn't need to react that way. I take full responsibility for my reaction." This exchange will bring you closer together and you will both be filled with love and foregiveness...and a mutual respect.

Experiencing and then letting go of anger by taking responsibility for it is a monumental step in your personal development. By taking it further and expressing it to the individual concerned, you will embrace a golden opportunity to show your love. This sharing exhibits a profound trust in your relationship on a very intimate level. It indicates that you have confidence in them and in your relationship enough to have the courage to open your heart completely.

If a similar situation occurs and you have learned to accept full responsibility for your reactions, you will no longer feel emotional. You will notice that, as you free yourself from the shackles of emotion, you will automatically let go of old grudges.

Perhaps you've been carrying the emotional baggage of unresolved conflict between yourself and siblings or friends. It was always "their fault". You've kept this all inside you - allowing it to fester and create a cellular sludge. LET IT GO! Take responsibility for what happened and what you are feeling and express it to them. You will not only experience an inner transformation when this is released, but you will notice physical changes as well - weight loss and a sense of lightness - a sense of well-being and inner satisfaction.

The energy center of emotion is located between the navel and the heart region. As we grow older, if we have accumulated a lot of emotional baggage, our waistline thickens. It is more common in men, as they "swallow" their emotions more than women do. They are not allowed to express them. In my workshops, I have witnessed thousands of people who have learned to master their emotions. The results are astounding! Letting go of the emotional baggage brought about an average loss of up to 15 centimeters in the waistline over a period of 2 - 3 months!

Many have regained their health and shed physical disease along with the emotional dis-ease. Many of them have freed themselves from cancer!

Once you have learned how to release yourself from emotional bondage, it will become clear that it can only be done with sincerity - from the heart. If you are expecting the other person to change after sharing your feelings with them, you are still using your mind instead of your heart. It takes courage to open your heart without expectations.

Here's an interesting little scenario: Let's pretend that it really bothers you when the kitchen cupboard doors are left open, but it doesn't bother anyone else in your household. You have two choices - you can react by saying: "No one cares enough about my feelings to shut the doors!" and feel angry, frustrated and put-upon by those "inconsiderate clods". OR... you can tell yourself: "I'm the one who likes them shut, so I will shut them." It takes less energy to shut the doors than it does to get upset. You have accepted responsibility for your emotions. From that moment on, you will stop being angry or frustrated. You may notice, however, that your family has begun to shut the cupboard doors, now that you have decided not to change their behavior.

Once you relax and accept responsibility for your own peace of mind, nothing is so intensely important anymore. Even if you disagree with something, it just won't affect you any longer. What a relief!

CHAPTER 18 EXERCISES

» Go through the process of expressing one emotion to someone else. You may choose to deal with one that you have been dragging around with you, to deal with one you are currently facing, or wait until a new one crops up. Believe me, a new one will crop up shortly. Be sure to express your emotion to this person AFTER you have taken responsibility for it. Acknowledge that you did not know how to love properly at the time.

» Practice the three steps in this chapter until you fully understand the process. You will enjoy a wonderful sense of well-being. You will see that it all comes back to the same thing: accept that love underlies every word and deed.

» Experiencing emotion indicates that you feel threatened in some way. Once you learn to live from the heart, to look through the eyes of love, you will master your emotions and they will never get the better of you again. You will automatically understand what lies behind the behavior of others.

» Here is your affirmation. Repeat it with sincerity until you feel it in your heart.

I ACCEPT ALL OF MY EMOTIONS AND I KNOW I HAVE THE POWER TO MASTER THEM BY ACCEPTING FULL RESPONSIBILITY FOR THEM. I NOW COMMUNICATE AND EXPRESS THEM FREELY.

CHAPTER 19

FEAR AND GUILT

Fear and guilt are the two most pervasive and pernicious human emotions. There is not one person who has never felt fear (which includes worry, by the way) at some time in his life.

Fear, like all emotions, is generated in the mind. Like truth, it is highly individual - what you fear may not be what someone else fears. Some people have fewer fears than others. They are called "brave". Others manage to overcome existing fears. If a large dog were to run toward you, the fear you may feel is very real. As far as you are concerned, you are in danger. However, to someone else who may have an affinity with animals, being approached by a large dog is an opportunity to befriend him. He is already convinced that the animal will not harm him. He understands that the dog is indicating that he wants to play.

It is important that you are aware of your fear so that you can determine whether or not it has justification. If your physical body is in danger, your fear is justified. Your body produces just the right amount of adrenaline required to face the given situation. How many times have you experienced fear over the past few months? Was your life really endangered? Was your fear real or imagined?

Recurring fears are the result of programming, or "imprinting" by your parents - perhaps as far back as your early childhood, or even before you were born. Overprotective parents unconsciously produce fear in their children. For example, a parent lives in constant fear that the baby will fall or catch cold, or pinch his fingers...etc. However common this habitual fear-based behavior is, it is not natural. As already discussed in this book, a person forms an image in his mind called an "elemental", which is fed unconsciously through thoughts and behavior that eventually cause it to materialize. REMEMBER:YOU ARE CONSTANTLY CREATING YOUR OWN REALITY!

This is why someone, living in constant fear of being robbed, gets robbed and why a woman, living in constant fear of being raped, gets raped. The more you fear something, even unconsciously, the more you make it happen. You consciously or unconsciously feed the situation in your mind until it has gained enough energy and momentum to manifest itself in reality.

Becoming conscious of what you are feeling or fearing will diffuse the energy that you would otherwise be channeling into making it happen. Through increased awareness and simple acts of love, you will be able to take a detached, objective look at your fears as they surface, without becoming emotionally attached to them. Thus, you will be in a position to master them.

Here's another example: Perhaps your parents left you for a period of time in unfamiliar surroundings when you were a small child. They may have taken a vacation and left you in the care of someone you didn't know or were uncomfortable with. You may have experienced strong feelings of rejection, even panic, at the possibility of never seeing your parents again. Finding the sense of rejection unbearable, you carry the fear of being rejected into your adult life. You are so afraid of rejection that you make it happen over and over. Whenever you get "too" close to someone, you unconsciously create circumstances through which you will be rejected.

The child who fears rejection gets rejected at school, at home and, in later life, will feel rejected by their spouse. Until they learn to master their fear or rejection, it will continue to happen. Fears operate subtly, breeding in the subconscious, producing other fears that gradually permeate the individual and develop into full-blown phobias.

There are many common, obvious fears such as: fear of the dark, of water, of tunnels, of bridges or elevators, of being stuck in a cramped space, fear of blushing (or showing emotion), of gaining weight, of lack of money, of animals, traffic, heights, depths, germs, crowds, death, sickness, accidents, fire, planes, cars, needles... and on and on.

There are just as many subtle fears such as: fear of not living up to someone's expectations, fear of being laughed at, rejected, abandoned, humiliated, criticized, accused, fear of hurting someone else's feelings...and more. The list is endless! Fear has a tremendous hold on us!

Those who exhibit the greatest number of fears often had parents who felt insecure and anxious themselves. Fearful parents breed fearful children. According to research done in the field, women exhibit more fears and phobias than men do.

A PHOBIA is a pronounced, chronic fear that usually rears its presence when major life changes occur. A possible sequence of such occurrences would be: the start of the school year, adolescence, adulthood, marriage, birth of a child, death of a spouse, divorce or even the death of someone close. During these critical times, a person's fears can become phobias.

According to recent research, the most common fears, by proportion, are as follows:

– 60%: Agoraphobia

– 20%: Disease or injury

– 10%: Death and crowds

– 5%: Animals

– 3%: Heights

– 2%: Other fears

As indicated, agoraphobia is the most prominent. What is it? Simply "the fear of fearing". I've had many opportunities to work with agoraphobics and must admit that this phobia is a difficult one to master at first and has a tremendous affect on the lives of the individuals who have it. Agoraphobia is not insurmountable, however -many people have freed themselves from its clutches.

The most difficult obstacle for the agoraphobic is the fact that they are dealing with two types of anxiety simultaneously. First, the situation itself, which scares them and secondly, the fact that others who do not understand or share their fear, think they're crazy, stupid or weak. For this reason, people with pronounced fears do their best to hide them, which is very damaging. In a close family environment the situation can be aggravated by an overprotective family member who goes along with the other's fears.

Agoraphobia culminates in the fear of being alone - away from familiar surroundings or reassuring people (i.e.: husband, wife, parents or even children). Usually the family home is the only place they feel secure. The moment they feel deprived of their outward security, fear invades them. They fear being alone in public, of losing consciousness, falling, having a heart attack...or of being ridiculed in front of others and being alone in the middle of a crowd. Their consummate fear is being alone.

In reality, usually nothing ever happens to them, but they exhibit physical symptoms of dizziness, great muscular tension or total lack of it, excessive perspiration, respiratory difficulties, nausea, urinary incontinence, palpitations and arrhythmia. If these symptoms occur when you are alone, you may be experiencing an attack of agoraphobia. Often, long-standing agoraphobics reach the point where they won't leave the house - even to go to the corner store. They fear "losing their grip", but never actually do. According to research in this field, women suffer more from phobias than men do.

*IMPORTANT: Accept that it is only a phobia - excessive and escalated fears that have been fed constantly with thoughts and energy. It is critical that the supply of thoughts and energy be cut off. The only solution is to look the fear in the eye and take action in spite of it. Start with small, daily victories. If you fear heights, start with a few steps at a time. If your fear is of animals, face small animals first - as your confidence grows, you can face larger ones. Regardless of the magnitude of the victory, you must congratulate yourself and let your family become involved and congratulate you on your victories too. FEAR IS NOT RATIONAL. Trying to over-come it rationally will not work. THE ONLY WAY TO DEAL WITH FEAR IS THROUGH DIRECT ACTION.

The employee who fears his boss but wants a raise will not have a chance of getting it hiding behind his desk. The only way is to take a deep breath, knock on the boss's door, face him and speak directly about what he wants. It is a good idea, also, to mention his fear. Ex-pressing it to others helps it become easier to master. It diffuses it and gives it an opening through which it can escape at its own rate.

Don't be afraid to admit fear! People who are trapped inside themselves and wrestling with their fears alone are perpetually tor-mented by them. An inner voice harasses them day and night. OPEN UP and you will see that your fears can be released slowly and easily, freeing you forever. Trying to avoid dealing with them through drugs or alcohol will only suppress them - they will return with a vengeance.

The moment you begin to feel frightened about something, ask yourself what you have to lose or to gain by submitting to the fear. If you are in the path of an oncoming truck, you have much to gain by feeling fear. The fear is real and justified in that case. Usually, though, fear is not advantageous and only cripples you in getting ahead. Facing and admitting your fear will give you a wonderful self-confidence that will carry over into every area of your life.

Because of fear, we tend to make the wrong decisions in a num-ber of situations. For example, you must decide between two activi-ties one evening. If you make your decision based on fear, you will inevitably make the wrong one.

Stay alert and conscious of how fear is affecting your life. If, for example, you accept an invitation only because you fear displeasing someone, you have made the wrong decision. Fear motivated you. If you are invited out but decide not to go because you are afraid of driving home in the dark, you have, once more, made the wrong de-cision. Being motivated by fear brings only disappointment and dis-satisfaction as you become slowly paralyzed and your self-esteem diminishes. Acknowledge the fear and you will be guided toward the right choices. You will learn to open up and go forward, knowing that the RIGHT decision is the one that is OPPOSITE to the fear-based decision.

The more you can learn to master you emotions, the less fearful you will become. Vibrations of fear are all around you and will penetrate unconsciously if you let them. Master your emotions and build a strong wall against fear. Agoraphobics are usually very sensitive, emotional people who leave themselves open to penetration by outside fears.

Imagine that your etheric, or subtle bodies form a beautiful, protective bubble around you. Pretend that the outer layer of that bubble is made up of all the energy from the fears you have mastered. For each fear that is not mastered, a flaw appears in the bubble, allowing a current of similar fears to seep in, disturbing your harmony. By using the powerful love that exists inside the bubble, the bubble itself is reinforced, repairing and healing any flaws. It becomes impenetrable. You will become immune to the invasion of destructive vibrations.

GUILT has become almost an art form in our culture - it is used to sell air time by the telephone companies and to manipulate family members and friends. It is one of the most powerful emotions!

"Feeling" guilty and "being" guilty are two very different things. Being guilty is knowing that you have intentionally hurt yourself or someone else. Take a hard look at yourself. When was the last time you INTENTIONALLY did harm to anyone? My guess is that it was a long time ago, if ever. Very few people are really guilty.

By understanding and accepting your innate inner perfection, you will begin to realize that you are free of fault; therefore free of guilt.

Intent is the key word. If, for example, you have insulted someone unintentionally, the other person may be angry and try to make you feel guilty. You say to yourself: "My God, I can't believe I said that to him!" Then ask yourself: "Am I guilty of doing this deliberately? Did I INTEND to hurt him?" If the answer is "no", you are not guilty.

There is no need to ask forgiveness or to feel guilty if you have done or said something unintentionally that may have hurt someone else (or yourself). If you are determined to feel guilty, your subconscious will punish you and will send you an "accident" signal. It is telling you that guilt is not beneficial to you.

If you have been hurt by someone else and seek revenge, you are guilty because you are acting consciously with the intent of bringing harm to him. You will cause an inner disturbance that will force you to admit guilt. In order to neutralize guilt, you must admit to your thoughts or actions and ask forgiveness from the other person or from yourself.

REMEMBER: every thought is a vibration that travels out into the world and is received by the person you are thinking of, whether he is aware of it or not. Whether the thought is one of love, or hatred, it will reach the one for whom it was intended.

You may have noticed that you are uncomfortable around certain people for no apparent reason. Outwardly, there is no discord, but there has been an inward exchange of negative energy that has caused an uneasiness between you. It is an indication that one or the other or even both of you are living contrary to the Law of Love.

In order to cleanse and purify your inner self, to love unconditionally, you must learn to rid yourself of each and every emotion as it arises. When you are guilty, address it and ask for forgiveness. Do if for your own sake, regardless of how you think the other person may react. Your ego, the inner voice that undermines your growth, will say: "What if he says?...what will he think of me...what if he makes fun of me... what if he accuses me...?" DON'T LISTEN.

Consider this scenario: A woman you know found that $20 was missing from her purse and jumped to the conclusion that you were the thief. On second thought, she realizes accusing you would be unfair. She approaches you and says: "You know, I had $20 disappear from my purse and I immediately thought you must have taken it. I can't believe I would have thought such a thing - can you forgive me?" What would you feel? Would you be angry with her? Certainly not! You would probably feel an overwhelming love and respect for her honesty and courage in being so open with you. When you communicate from the heart, you will instantly be understood by the heart of another. This is love's natural law: HEART TO HEART, not heart to head or head to head.

Listen carefully to yourself. Are you constantly giving excuses? There is a saying: "Someone who excuses himself, accuses himself". Are you guilty?

If you break a glass while doing the dishes, how do you react? Think about it - did you break it on purpose? Perhaps just for the fun of it? Not likely. Why are you so hard on yourself? An accident is brought on by your subconscious - it is the way you punish yourself to neutralize guilt. Ask yourself what you were feeling guilty about and deal with it. Stop blaming yourself; learn to love and accept yourself and you will do the same for others easily.

Are you the type of person who feels guilt toward yourself? Are you self-critical? How often do you accuse yourself unfairly, called yourself names and felt "like an idiot" for having forgotten something? Would you treat your best friend that way or would you be more gentle, more forgiving of him? YOU ARE YOUR BEST FRIEND! Have you forgotten? Forgive yourself. Accept yourself and know that you are doing your best. Once you learn to treat yourself with love and kindness, you will do the same for others. It will become much easier to see their perfection.

CHAPTER 19 EXERCISES

» Identify all of your fears. Choose to master one of them and take action, one step at a time. Do the same for all of the fears you have listed.

» Make a list of all the things you felt guilty about over the past three days. Beside each one, note whether you were actually guilty or whether you just "felt guilty".

» Note any accidents over the past week and determine what you were feeling guilty about at the time.

» Repeat the following affirmation often until the little voice in your head stops and until you stop feeding all your energy to the fears you have created. No matter how long you have felt worried, doubtful or tormented, this affirmation will apply:

I AM THE SOLE MASTER OF MY LIFE AND ANY CONSCIENCE WITHIN ME, OTHER THAN MY OWN, IS EXPELLED AND RELEASED IMMEDIATELY.

The more energy you put into this affirmation (rather than just thinking it), the more impact it will have and the faster the results. Say it out loud in front of the mirror, if need be.

In this affirmation, "another consciousness" is mentioned. I am referring to the little voices that undermine your true self - the ones that are born of insecurity and fed by fear. Refuse to listen to them any longer and they will die out. You will no longer feed them.

For the person who is wrestling with chronic fears and phobias, I strongly suggest that you say this affirmation hundreds, if not thousands, of times a day, to flush out the negative energies. After a few weeks, you will feel lighter and the battle will become easier. YOU CAN OVERCOME!

CHAPTER 20

EMOTIONAL ESSENTIALS

To maintain optimal emotional health, there are seven fundamental needs that must be met. They are discussed here in order of importance. The more nourishment you give to your emotional body, the closer you will get to mastering your emotions.

BEAUTY as seen through the inner and the outer eye, beauty that is heart-felt nourishes the soul. It calms the mind and relaxes the physical body. Beauty vibrates on a higher plane than what is ugly or mundane. I'm sure you are familiar with the "high" that you experience when something you see has really moved you and touched your soul. You sense a deep feeling of peace and happiness, as if all is right with the world, if only for a moment.

As the saying goes: "Beauty is in the eye of the beholder." In other words, as in any other reality, it is determined by your perception. When you live from the heart, you see love and beauty in everything and everyone. In those who are spiritually advanced, this results in a state of bliss.

On a more basic level, one's environment is a determining factor in his emotional health. People who are sad or seriously ill usually are unable to see beauty around or within them. One who is surrounded by ugliness - perhaps living within barren concrete walls, deprived of any natural influence (trees, grass, flowers, etc.), will find his own vibration depleted. He will begin to neglect his own physical appearance and have suicidal tendencies. It is difficult to visualize beauty for any length of time, when surrounded by ugliness.

Take a walk in the park, in the woods or near water. The profound beauty that nature exhibits provides nourishment for your emotional body. Consciously try to "become one" with a sunset, a tree, and observe your body's reaction on every level -physically, mentally, emotionally and spiritually.

Every moment and every circumstance in your life offers you an opportunity to experience beauty. Take in as much of it as you can - until your heart is full. In this way, your life will also become fuller and richer. Start simply with the food you ingest and the clothes you wear. Choose quality rather than quantity. Remember that your skin is your body's largest organ and that it is extremely sensitive to what it comes in contact with! Be sure that you wear natural fibers as much as possible, as many man-made fibers are petroleum and chemical-based. Your body actually absorbs these poisons through your skin. The dyes in some fabrics are also toxic to the body. Be sure your clothes are comfortable and make you feel good, allowing your vibration to come through.

Become acutely aware of beauty around you and decide NOW to make it a priority whenever you are choosing a new home or making a purchase of any kind. Accept and acknowledge your own inner and outer beauty and accept all compliments without saying anything derogatory about yourself in response to them.

Respiratory and heart problems are indications that you are stifling the life-force around you and refusing to see the beauty in all life.

CREATIVITY is the expression of your individuality, your essential nature. Lack of creative expression in your life will affect your well-being. If you are currently trapped in a job that is monotonous or unfulfilling, you must compensate with creative recreation until you can find a job that will inspire you. If your work requires you to be creative, you may want to balance it with a more mundane life at home.

Everyone, regardless of gender, health, cultural background, age or economic status, can and must create. You don't have to invent anything or paint another Mona Lisa, but something as simple as preparing dinner can give you the satisfaction that any creative endeavor provides. Leave your mark wherever you go and use your own personal touch when decorating or doing repairs around your home.

Everyone has special talents and abilities that are uniquely theirs. Look back into your childhood. Did you enjoy writing or drawing? People are usually good at what they enjoy doing most. Take the time to draw, or take a watercolor or woodworking class for pure enjoyment. You will be surprised how it will open you up. Don't worry if what you are producing is "marketable" or how anyone else will feel about it. DO IT FOR YOURSELF! I know many people who have "always dreamed of writing a book". If you are one of those people, start writing it - purely for your own growth and enjoyment.

It is very common for people to be afraid to express their creativity. "What if so-and-so doesn't like it?..What if I don't think it's good enough?" LET GO AND LET IT GO! Be yourself - express yourself and your quality of life will improve dramatically! As discussed in Chapter 12, your creativity is closely aligned with your sexuality. Diminished creative expression will directly affect the throat and sexual organs. CREATE YOUR LIFE NOW!

CONFIDENCE, in this context, refers to self-confidence, which is the capacity to express and reveal oneself to another without fear of being judged.

Confidence is often misinterpreted as courage, perseverance and audacity. The truly self-confident person trusts and has faith in his innate perfection; thus he has no fear of exposing imperfection. His openness attracts other people's trust. Others open up to him because they know that, as he does not judge himself, he will not judge them.

Most people choose to open up to specific people about specific areas of their lives. They wouldn't think to open up about their personal problems to an employer, or about their sexual problems to a friend, for example. The self-confident person uses his discretion, but is comfortable with almost anyone. Being in tune with his essence, he is usually correct in assessing whether or not another person is able to handle the openness.

Remember that "employers" are other human beings, with lives of their own. Opening up to them gives them the message that you are the type of person who "lays his cards on the table". This will generate trust and a strong working relationship.

Most people refuse to open up to each other out of fear of judgment. If you feel an urge to confide in someone, even though you may not know them well, go ahead and do it. Your intuition is spurring you on to connect with others.

You can choose to be self-confident. It is not a hereditary characteristic. Through willingness and positive action, you will learn to reveal yourself. Lack of self-confidence causes you to "hide" who you are - this brings about a lack of trust from others.

Failing to "open up and let go" in terms of your personality, manifests physically in the organs of elimination, i.e.: the kidneys, skin and bowels.

BELONGING is defined as a sense of being "part of" something...a group, a community, a family... It validates us and gives us a sense of order. Some people are in tune enough with the Universe to understand and acknowledge their place in it. Most of us just want to "find our place in this world." Where do we "belong"?

People who have no sense of belonging feel 'lost' and become withdrawn, isolating themselves even further. You must understand that this sense of belonging must come from within you. It is entirely up to you whether or not you want to become involved in life - you decide if and when you will belong to something, someone and when.

If you habitually go to the same restaurant, the same vacation spot or spend time with the same group of friends , it indicates that your sense of belonging is not well-developed. You feel a need to hang on to what is familiar to you and are uncomfortable in new environments. You have yet to understand that the world belongs to everyone and that your place is wherever you want it to be. Nowhere are you excluded. It is all up to you.

"Belonging" somewhere does not mean, necessarily , that you want to live there, but wherever you are at any given time (whether among the poor or the wealthy), you have the right to be there at that moment. By understanding and accepting this concept, you will learn to be comfortable anywhere.

People who have a poorly-developed sense of belonging often try to fill their emptiness with food or alcohol. They usually have weight or digestive problems. They can become possessive with other people to compensate for their feeling of not belonging.

HOPE is that "light at the end of tunnel" - that you've heard about. If you were actually trapped in an underground tunnel with no exit and were convinced there was no chance you would ever get out, you would feel you had no reason to stay alive. What for? You're going to die in there anyway, right? Imagine this situation clearly in your mind until you can feel the hopelessness and feel your "flame go out." Suddenly, you realize that there is a small pin-point of light peeking through somewhere deep down in the tunnel. You immediately feel a resurgence of energy and life. THAT IS HOPE. Regardless of any obstacle you may encounter - digging your way out of that tunnel, you know there's a way out! You will move toward the light - toward freedom!

Realize in your everyday life that everything turns out for the best. There is a Divine Plan, even though you may not see or under-stand it, there is a bigger picture. Whatever you are experiencing right now is part of your development; it is a learning experience. As you go forward and grow, there will be more light, more warmth, more love - inside you and in your life. DON'T EVER LOSE HOPE! Those who have lost hope experience depression and/or low blood pressure as their flame burns low.

AFFECTION is expressed through physical contact, words of encouragement, gifts, flowers, notes, compliments, small deeds (or large ones) or simply, a warm smile. With affection, you "affect" someone else. If you are lacking affection in your life, did you forget to sow some?

People often find that it is easier to give affection to their pets than to other human beings. Often you will see one spouse sitting in front of the television set, petting his dog or cat, while the other spouse is left alone, resigned to satisfying his own needs. When you withdraw your affection, you create barriers in your relationships.

A friend of mine told me that, since her dog died, she and her husband and daughter were much more affectionate toward each other. It had never occurred to them that they had been directing all their affection toward the dog and neglecting each other.

Remember, on the earth plane, energy is at the root of everything. What you put into something in terms of energy, is what you will get out of it. It may grow from what you put in therefore reaping even more, but it will never diminish in its return. The more you allow the energy of your affection to circulate, the more will come back to you. Research has shown that babies who have only their basic needs met (food, diapering, etc.) but who are given no affection, can actually die! WE MUST CONNECT with each other!

People often say "yes" when they mean "no" because they need the attention of others, or their "affection". We have a need to affect other people and have them affect us. Human interaction is vital. The best way to interact is to offer your help and guidance, your affection, without expectations. Then the flow will not be interrupted.

If you feel you have no affect on the lives of others but your environment affects you, you will create a terrible imbalance in your body. Your flow of energy will become stuck and you will become withdrawn and even more isolated. Get in touch with what you are feeling - express it - show your love and "warm up"!

If you block the affection (giving and receiving) in your life, you will experience allergies and the same physical problems that you will experience without a sense of belonging, as they are closely tied.

GOALS are critical! They give you a reason to get up in the morning - a purpose. If I were to ask you to take only one minute and tell me your short-term goals (6 months), mid-range goals (5 years) and long-range goals (20 years), what would you tell me? Could you list three in each category? It would be difficult -especially if they don't exist!

Without goals, the energy of your life becomes stagnant - it stops flowing because you have no place for it to go! Goals will increase the quality of your life by giving it life! Have specific goals - even grand ones. IT IS BETTER TO MISS A GREAT GOAL BY A LITTLE THAN TO ACHIEVE A SMALL ONE.

Don't be afraid to set goals - you can change them. If you decide to learn French within six months and decide a month into it that you would prefer to learn Spanish, switch! Just make sure you keep going forward.

Be sure you understand the difference between goals and desires. Goals start with a desire; taking action turns them into goals. If, for example, you desire a house. That house will become a goal the moment you start taking action toward getting it. Put your energy into achieving it - start clipping newspaper ads, visiting open houses, getting a "feel" for the market, mentally decorating the interior and putting money aside.

If I told you to start putting even $10 a week aside for a big project like buying a house, you would tell me I was crazy. "What kind of impact would $10 a week have on buying a house? That would take forever!" The point is, it's a step in the right direction - you are telling your subconscious mind to start driving toward your dream!

A large number of people live alone. Most of them would like to meet "the perfect mate", but make no effort in that direction. Instead, they live their lives through television, ignoring their own lives. How do they expect to meet their perfect mate? Take action - start talking to and meeting people every day. Your mate is out there somewhere.

A dream becomes a reality when you turn it into a goal. You will be filled with energy and a strong sense of purpose. Be careful not to be too rigid - maintain your flexibility. You will need it, as the road to your goal will not be perfectly straight. As you travel along it, you may encounter more beneficial options. Keep your eyes and ears open and keep an open mind. If you change your mind about a goal or project , don't let the opinions of others pressure you into continuing.

When you decide to turn a desire into a goal, rather than discuss it with other people (especially those who scare easily and who will do their best to talk you out of it), consult your superconscious mind. It will give you signals as to whether or not your dream is in your best interest.

Without goals, without a purpose, you will lack energy. You will feel depressed, lethargic and apathetic. You may begin to have problems with your legs, arms, eyes, ears and nose.

CHAPTER 20 EXERCISES

» Before continuing onto Chapter 21, take a sheet of paper and write down the needs of your emotional body.

» Determine which of these needs you have been neglecting. Which emotional nutrients do you need?

» Once you learn to meet your emotional needs and nurture your emotional body, you will begin to master your emotions and MASTER YOUR LIFE!

» Here is your affirmation:

I AM NOW DETERMINED TO RESPECT THE NEEDS OF MY EMOTIONAL BODY AND I REGAIN MY EMOTIONAL HEALTH.

PART FIVE:

SPIRITUALITY AND MEDITATION

CHAPTER 21

HARMONY AND BALANCE

The truly spiritual being understands that others are mirrors of himself. This is a profound and extraordinary revelation that becomes the lifeline to your personal development. As you grow in your awareness of this concept, you will begin to see that the more love and beauty you see outside of yourself, the more love and beauty will be reflected within you. A sense of peace overcomes you once you truly understand and accept that everything and everyone is "as it should be". Can you imagine what this world would be like if we could all see the God-self, the perfection, in each other?

The smallest criticism or the slightest judgment toward another is a reflection of what you judge and do not accept about yourself. When you criticize or judge someone, it's as though you were saying: "I am GOD and the other is not" A truly spiritual person sees his own perfection, his God-self as clearly as he sees the perfection in others. We are all manifestations of God, but we must learn to express God as a whole.

Beethoven's ninth symphony is a masterpiece of creative genius. It is the expression of Beethoven's God-self, thus it resonates with the God-self within each of us, elevating our vibrations to a level of blissful union. I'm sure you have experienced the transcendent moment that happens when you are "one with the music" -when it has touched your soul.

If an amateur musician performs it, the symphony is expressed according to his limited ability. However, regardless of his level of expertise, the symphony itself remains inspired. As the musician learns to express it more fully, he will move closer and closer to its perfection. This takes practice, perseverance and a sense of purpose and dedication on his part, but is dependent primarily on his openness to the message in the music. The reason we are on this planet is to learn to express Divine Perfection and we will do it in our own way - our own style - at our own pace.

When our souls were conceived, we were each given a puzzle that was identical to the puzzle given to all. Since each of us is unique, we will put the puzzle together in our own way. Some will do it more quickly than others, some will start with the edge, some according to color: most of us will grab what we can identify with at random. Ultimately, to complete our evolution, we must complete our puzzle.

To criticize and judge the way others are putting their puzzles together takes time and energy away from your own. How can you possibly determine whether someone else is "doing it right"? If we would only learn from each other, we could put all of our puzzles together more easily.

Using the mirror analogy, you begin to understand any reaction you have to what you are seeing in others is because you do not accept the same thing in yourself. It strikes a chord in you because you identify with it, whether it is a behavior or a personality trait. Your superconscious mind is giving you a signal that whatever is bothering you about someone else is something you need to identify and work on in yourself. You do not allow that part of you to be seen because at some point in your life you had decided that such a trait was unacceptable. You no longer acknowledge who you are. Once you have learned to respect yourself, you will be able to accept others. Like a mirror, seeing beauty in others is a reflection of your own inner beauty. Express the beauty that is yours.

So, instead of judging the behavior of others and reacting to it, accept the fact this personality trait is in you and ask yourself what the consequences would be if you were to act the same way. What do you have to gain by behaving differently? Concentrate on your own puzzle - by concerning yourself with everyone else's, you will be neglecting your own. GET IT TOGETHER! The more puzzles that are completed, the closer our world will be to perfection!

If someone asks you for help, do your best to give it to them. We are here to grow together, but be sure the door is open before you allow yourself to go in. If you feel the urge to help someone, ask their permission first. Say: "I have something important to tell you, which I truly believe could help you now. Would it be all right if I shared it with you? " or "May I offer my opinion? I think I have something valuable to offer you that could help you in this situation." They may be very grateful to have your help with their puzzle, but if they prefer to do it themselves, respect their wishes.

By learning to see Divine Perfection in everyone and everything around you, your life will be transformed. You will feel you are constantly bathed in energy.

All life forms in the entire Universe are Divine expressions of God. Every living thing has an innate understanding of Divine Law - only mankind has lost touch with this and has a need to re-learn it.

Living "in the moment" is a characteristic of the spiritually evolved human being. That becomes increasingly difficult to do as the pace of our world increases. All most of us can do is "hang on" - so many of us choose to "hang on" to the past. By hanging on to the past, you are hanging on to accumulated, outdated thoughts and possessions that drag you down and slow you down. It's like climbing a staircase, taking each stair and piling it on your shoulders as you go . What a terrible burden you place on yourself! Are you hanging onto your past? Take a look around your home. Are your closets, your drawers, your attic and your basement crammed with accumulated "stuff"? Do you hesitate to get rid of all that "stuff"? Ask yourself what you are REALLY hanging onto and learn to let it go.

Now that you have decided to clean your "inner house", do some real housecleaning as well. Gather up all the stuff you haven't used in a year and give it away. Begin to circulate the energy that you have been hoarding so that it no longer clogs your life. The more you can let go and let the energy circulate, the more you will free up your own energy and attract new energy to you. Energy that is not in motion is misused. This is the simple Law of Emptiness (one of the fundamental Laws of Prosperity)- to create space for new things and ideas.

While many people remain attached to the past, some think only of the future. They either worry about it or wait for things to happen to them. "When I get married, my life will be better...when I get a house...when I have a child...when I lose weight..." Life is happening NOW! You are alive NOW! BE HAPPY, BE YOURSELF -NOW and everything will come to you. Your energy must be focused on NOW in order to take action.

Learn to think in this order: 1. BEING 2. DOING 3. HAVING, instead of "having, doing and then being." If you are the type of person that says "If I could HAVE this, then I could DO that, then I would BE happy...", you will never have, do or be anything. That way of thinking is in reverse to the necessary process. Here's an example of effective thinking: "BE HAPPY, DO WHAT YOU WANT AND YOU WILL GET WHAT YOU WANT"

The New Age is only beginning - it is based on the philosophy of BEING, rather than HAVING. All those who persist in thinking that "having" is more important than "being", will continue to be unfulfilled. Getting rid of everything you own is not the answer. The answer lies in LETTING GO of your attachment to things and old ideas. LET GO AND LET GROW so that you can focus on being happy, which is NOW!

Don't waste your time worrying about the future. Concentrate on NOW and have faith in your own ability and the Universal Law of Abundance to ensure that you will be provided for. You become what you think - you create your reality. Gather your resources, stand tall and find your balance. BE YOURSELF, in all your perfection, and everything will be as it should. Then you can go forward in confidence, toward your goals and the realization of your dreams!

Trust your innate divinity to guide you. Know that, when something "unpleasant" happens, that it is a necessary learning experience for you. It is a signal from your superconscious mind that you are thinking, speaking or acting in a manner contrary to the Law of Love. It is a little nudge from your God-self that helps to keep you on track. Operate from your heart center at all times and only good things will happen in your life.

Meditation will help you by quieting your mind so that you can hear the inner voice of your Superconscious mind. This is essential to your evolution. Meditate daily so that you can build a clear and open channel of communication with your God-self - your best friend and your guide.

Meditation is not a "relaxation"; it is a focused stillness of the mind. It is a gathering of your energies that are otherwise scattered. By bringing them all to one place, you create an antenna to the Divine.

Set aside 20 - 30 minutes a day, preferably early in the morning before breakfast. If this is not possible, at least try to meditate on an empty stomach - the process of digestion is very distracting and your vibration will be higher if your stomach is empty.

Be sure to find a quiet spot where you can be alone, undisturbed. If possible, choose a place with an eastern window, facing the rising sun. Sit with a straight back , with your feet flat on the floor so that the energy can flow freely from the base of your spine to the top of your head. Peaceful music may be used, if it will help shut out the outside world. Repeat a sentence or a simple word, called a "Mantra" that will help you to gather your thoughts to one place. Try to find a word that does not conjure up an image to which you have no specific visual association, such as "peace, love or harmony". The mantra we recommend in my workshops is "I AM GOD, GOD I AM". The more you repeat these words the more you will help your subconscious find the means to express them in your life.

If may be difficult, at first, to let go - to stop thinking. Persevere and it will pay off. Just as it would be in a physical training program, the initial pain and clumsiness gradually subsides. After a few days, or weeks, or a month, you will find you won't want to do without it.

In meditation, you will learn to switch off your mind and to listen to the voice of your Superconscious mind. It becomes a beautiful, intimate time that is deeply personal to you. Answers will be provided to you pertaining to your inner questions, not necessarily during the meditation, but during the following hours or days. If, during meditation, you experience physical discomfort anywhere in your body, simply acknowledge it and observe it. It will go away on its own, as you relax and accept it.

You will feel a love for your body and a oneness with it that you would never have imagined. You will begin to understand that it houses your soul and you will be grateful for it and will automatically take better care of it. It will begin to release accumulated stress. Thank your body for letting it go.

CHAPTER 21 EXERCISES

» List some of the behaviors that bother you in other people.

» Which of these behaviors do you recognize in yourself? You may be very surprised, if you are honest with yourself.

» Accept these behaviors in yourself and as you do so, ask yourself: "What does it cost me to behave this way? What am I gaining from it?"

» Make a second list of the things you admire in others.

» Which of these traits do you possess? Accept that you own these traits and understand that you deserve them. Give yourself permission to be as talented and as wonderful as the person you admire.

» Take as much time as you need to discover yourself, your abilities and your talents. Embark on this journey of discovery with an open mind and a sense of self-love and acceptance.

» REMEMBER: You are a manifestation of God. Nothing else exists but this Divine Perfection!

» Here is your affirmation. Note that it is the same as the affirmation at the end of Chapter One. Is there a difference between how you feel about it now compared to how you did after reading Chapter One?

I AM A MANIFESTATION OF THE DIVINE, I AM GOD AND I CREATE WHATEVER I DESIRE. KNOWING THIS, I FEEL A GREAT INNER STRENGTH AND A PROFOUND INNER PEACE.

CONCLUSION

You are on this earth for one purpose: to evolve, to grow, to accept the Divine Perfection in yourself and in others.

We return to this earth plane many times to deal with a variety of circumstances. It enlarges our frame of reference by experiencing different lives. Only in doing so do we learn how to love unconditionally.

Life is a great privilege, an opportunity to attend the school of love that is the earthly experience. Each moment is precious here, so live your life to the fullest. Do your utmost in each lifetime and you will reach your spiritual goals quickly and less painfully. It works the same way as in a regular school: if you waste your time and refuse to learn, you will have to return over and over again until you get it right.

The time spent "between lives" can be compared to summer vacation. Near the end of your vacation, you become excited about the prospect of a "clean slate". You vow to keep your notebooks tidy, to do all your homework, to "make this year your best ever!" You are anxious to get started. Once you are back in school, you lose sight of your goals and your good intentions become weak. Many of you find this is your experience in the earth school.

Some students, on the other hand, advance very quickly and remain eager and enthusiastic throughout their education. They may even skip several grades in the process. Their inner peace is attained much sooner. What kind of student are you? It's up to you to decide and to change at any time.

Once you learn to see God, or Divine Perfection, in everyone and everything around you, everything else falls into place. Beauty will be everywhere, in everything. You will love and accept each person just as they are now. Your fears will vanish and all negative emotions will disappear. You will no longer be a slave to your ego and you will enjoy glowing good health and happiness, whether in your relationships with others or with yourself. You will experience prosperity everywhere and on every level -in your physical and in your spiritual life.

The more you express your inner God by loving yourself and others, the more your inner light will radiate outward to the rest of the world. You will become a source of light, love and service to others - you will become God's gift to whoever is lucky enough to touch your life.

With all my heart I wish for you a life that is full and rich, that you may enjoy it with others. May you finally experience the peace and happiness that you truly deserve.

Who wants to enjoy life?

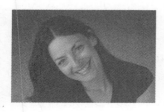

The dynamic and powerful teachings of the "Listen to Your Body" workshop are aimed at all people who are interested in **enjoying their life**. For the past 25 years, this workshop has provided participants with a vital source of knowledge as well as a solid foundation for being in harmony with themselves. Year after year, the startling results and enriching transformations achieved by over 40,000 people who have attended this workshop are truly astounding. **Those who read her books were surprised to see how much further the workshop brought them.**

Improve the quality of your life in just 2 days!

- ► Are you happy?
- ► Do you often feel guilty?
- ► Is disappointment part of your life?
- ► Do you get along with people easily?
- ► Are you full of energy?
- ► Do you have the life you want?
- ► Is it difficult for you to say no?
- ► Do you need to be perfect before loving yourself?

Come and see how our workshop can help you!

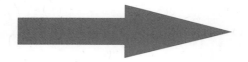

Stop putting up with your problems!

Thanks to this workshop, thousands of people are no longer putting up with life - they are living it! They have regained control over their lives and are using the wealth of personal power within them to create the lives they really want. The rewards are far greater than could be imagined.

The "Listen to Your Body" workshop has tangible effects at all levels: physical, emotional, mental and spiritual.

What do people think?

"Thanks for filling my heart and giving me new tools!"

"Thank you so much for a wonderful weekend. I look forward to growing!"

"It has been a delight and an honor to spend this time with you. Thank you for all the insights, the education and the fun! I wish you all the best."

"It has been a wonderful experience!"

"Thank you for sharing your wisdom... you inspire me."

"Thanks for a great weekend. The info will last a lifetime and improve it as I walk the path."

"Thank you for the light you shone on my path. The future reserves many nice surprises and I have the impression that your light will be part of it."

Visit our website or call us

To find out when and where the next workshop will be held.

1-888-437-8382 or 450-431-5336
www.listentoyourbody.net

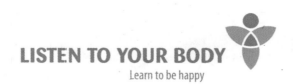

LISTEN TO YOUR BODY

Learn to be happy

Don't miss a thing!

Subscribe today to receive our bi-monthly newsletter including advice from Lise

It's easy!

Visit our website and fill in the subscription window on our home page

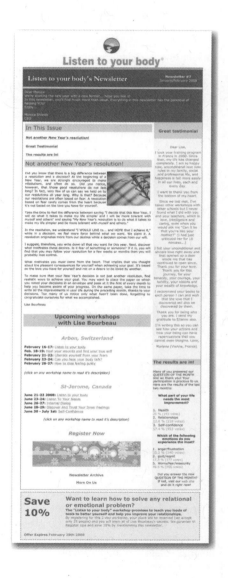

www.listentoyourbody.net

Books from the same author

Listen to your best friend on Earth, your body

LISE BOURBEAU takes you by the hand and, step by step, leads you beyond "packing your own parachute", to taking that step back into the clear, refreshing stream of life that flows from the Universal Source. She gives you the tools, not only to fix what is wrong in your life, but to build a solid foundation for your inner house - a foundation that extends as far as the global village. In this book, she helps you build an intimate, rewarding and powerful relationship with the most important person in your life - yourself.

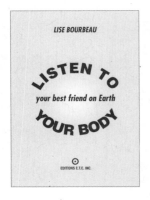

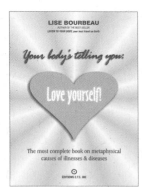

Your body's telling you: Love yourself!

Lise Bourbeau has compiled 20 years of research in the field of metaphysics and it's physical manifestations in the body and brought it all to the forefront in this user-friendly reference guide, Your body's telling you: Love yourself! Since 1982, she has worked successfully with over 15,000 people, helping them to unearth the underlying causes of specific illnesses and diseases.

"I am certain that any physical problem is simply the outward manifestation of dis-ease on psychological and/or emotional levels. The physical body is responding to this imbalance and warning of the need to return to the path of love and harmony."

Cover to cover, the reader discovers a most powerful tool, as he becomes his own healer. The reference material, a comprehensive guide to the causes of over 500 illnesses and diseases, is a succinct and visionary work that is truly and literally a labor of love.

Heal your wounds and find your true self

Do you sometimes feel that you are going around in circles in your personal growth? Do you occasionally see a problem re-emerge, thinking you had solved it? Perhaps it's because you're not looking in the right place.

This new book by Lise Bourbeau, as concrete as her others, demonstrates that all problems, whether physical, emotional or mental, stem from five important wounds: *rejection, abandonment, humiliation, betrayal* and *injustice*. This book contains detailed descriptions of these wounds and of the masks we've developed to hide them.

This book will allow you to set off on the path that leads to complete healing, the path that leads to your ultimate goal: your true self.

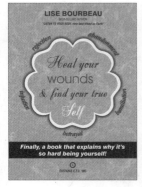

4 ways to order

TITLE	QTY.	TOTAL
SUB-TOTAL		
SHIPPING		
TOTAL		

info@listentoyourbody.net

450-431-0991

ECOUTE TON CORPS
1102 La Salette Blv
St-Jerome (Quebec)
J5L 2J7   CANADA

1-800-361-3834
or 450-431-5336

SHIPPING & HANDLING FEES
CANADA: 8.50$can
US: 10$can
INTERNATIONAL: contact us

VISA

Number: _____ Exp.: __ / __
month   year

Cardholder's name: _____

MasterCard

Signature: _____

☐ **CANADIAN MONEY ORDER made out to ECOUTE TON CORPS**

Name: _____

Address: _____

City/Town: _____   Zip code: _____

Telephone #: (___) _____

The production of this title on Rolland Enviro 100 Print paper instead of virgin fibres paper reduces your ecological footprint by :

Tree(s) : 27
Solid waste : 1 494 kg
Water : 98 649 L
Air emissions : 3 884 kg

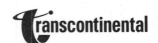

    100% PERMANENT

Printed on Rolland Enviro 100, containing 100 % post-consumer recycled fibers, Eco-Logo certified, Processed without chlorinate, FSC Recycled and manufactured using biogas energy.